Controversies in Rheumatology

Editors

JONATHAN KAY
SERGIO SCHWARTZMAN

RHEUMATIC DISEASE CLINICS OF NORTH AMERICA

www.rheumatic.theclinics.com

Consulting Editor
MICHAEL H. WEISMAN

August 2019 • Volume 45 • Number 3

ELSEVIER

1600 John F. Kennedy Boulevard • Suite 1800 • Philadelphia, Pennsylvania, 19103-2899
http://www.theclinics.com

RHEUMATIC DISEASE CLINICS OF NORTH AMERICA Volume 45, Number 3
August 2019 ISSN 0889-857X, ISBN 13: 978-0-323-69828-3

Editor: Lauren Boyle
Developmental Editor: Casey Potter

Rheumatic Disease Clinics of North America (ISSN 0889-857X) is published quarterly by Elsevier Inc., 360 Park Avenue South, New York, NY 10010-1710. Months of issue are February, May, August, and November. Business and editorial offices: 1600 John F. Kennedy Boulevard, Suite 1800, Philadelphia, PA 19103-2899. Periodicals postage paid at New York, NY and additional mailing offices. Subscription prices are USD 362.00 per year for US individuals, USD 706.00 per year for US institutions, USD 100.00 per year for US students and residents, USD 427.00 per year for Canadian individuals, USD 925.00 per year for Canadian institutions, USD 465.00 per year for international individuals, USD 925.00 per year for international institutions, and USD 230.00 per year for Canadian and foreign students/residents. To receive student/resident rate, orders must be accompanied by name of affiliated institution, date of term, and the *signature* of program/residency coordinator on institution letterhead. Orders will be billed at individual rate until proof of status received. Foreign air speed delivery is included in all *Clinics* subscription prices. All prices are subject to change without notice. **POSTMASTER:** Send address changes to *Rheumatic Disease Clinics of North America,* Elsevier Health Sciences Division, Subscription Customer Service, 3251 Riverport Lane, Maryland Heights, MO 63043. **Customer Service: 1-800-654-2452 (US and Canada). From outside of the US and Canada: 314-447-8871. Fax: 314-447-8029. For print support, e-mail: JournalsCustomerService-usa@elsevier.com**. **For online support, e-mail: JournalsOnline Support-usa@elsevier.com**.

Reprints. For copies of 100 or more of articles in this publication, please contact the Commercial Reprints Department, Elsevier Inc., 360 Park Avenue South, New York, New York, 10010-1710; Tel.: +1-212-633-3874, Fax: +1-212-633-3820, and E-mail: reprints@elsevier.com.

Rheumatic Disease Clinics of North America is covered in *MEDLINE/PubMed (Index Medicus), Current Contents/Clinical Medicine, Science Citation Index, ISI/BIOMED,* and *EMBASE/Excerpta Medica.*

Contributors

CONSULTING EDITOR

MICHAEL H. WEISMAN, MD
Distinguished Professor of Medicine Emeritus, David Geffen School of Medicine at UCLA, Professor of Medicine Emeritus, Cedars-Sinai Medical Center, Los Angeles, California, USA

EDITORS

JONATHAN KAY, MD
Professor, Department of Medicine and Population and Quantitative Health Sciences, Timothy S. and Elaine L. Peterson Chair in Rheumatology, Director of Clinical Research, Rheumatology, UMass Memorial Medical Center and University of Massachusetts Medical School, Worcester, Massachusetts, USA

SERGIO SCHWARTZMAN, MD
Franchellie M. Cadwell Associate Professor of Medicine, Hospital for Special Surgery, New York Presbyterian Hospital, Weill Medical College of Cornell University, New York, New York, USA

AUTHORS

DANIEL ALBERT, MD
Professor, Department of Medicine and Pediatrics, The Dartmouth Institute, Geisel School of Medicine, Dartmouth-Hitchcock Medical Center, Hanover, New Hampshire, USA

DANIEL ALETAHA, MD
Division of Rheumatology, Department of Internal Medicine 3, Medical University, Vienna, Austria

PAMELA BAGLEY, PhD, MSLIS
Biomedical Libraries, Dartmouth College, Hanover, New Hampshire, USA

JOEL A. BLOCK, MD
Department of Internal Medicine, Division of Rheumatology, Rush University Medical Center, Chicago, Illinois, USA

LAURA C. COATES, MB ChB, MRCP, PhD
NIHR Clinician Scientist, Nuffield Department of Orthopaedics, Rheumatology and Musculoskeletal Sciences, Botnar Research Centre, Oxford, United Kingdom

JONATHAN KAY, MD
Professor, Department of Medicine and Population and Quantitative Health Sciences, Timothy S. and Elaine L. Peterson Chair in Rheumatology, Director of Clinical Research, Rheumatology, UMass Memorial Medical Center and University of Massachusetts Medical School, Worcester, Massachusetts, USA

C. KENT KWOH, MD
Chief, Division of Rheumatology, Director, University of Arizona Arthritis Center, University of Arizona College of Medicine, Tucson, Arizona, USA

WALTER P. MAKSYMOWYCH, MD, FRCP(C)
Professor, Department of Medicine, Division of Rheumatology, University of Alberta, Edmonton, Alberta, Canada

NANCY OLSEN, MD
Chief, Division of Rheumatology, Professor, Department of Medicine, Penn State M.S. Hershey Medical Center, Hershey, Pennsylvania, USA

ANNA PLAAS, PhD
Department of Internal Medicine, Division of Rheumatology, Rush University Medical Center, Chicago, Illinois, USA

HANI RASHID, DO
Fellow, Division of Rheumatology, University of Arizona College of Medicine, Tucson, Arizona, USA

CARRIE RICHARDSON, MD, MHS
Department of Internal Medicine, Division of Rheumatology, Rush University Medical Center, Chicago, Illinois, USA

KENNETH G. SAAG, MD, MSc
Jane Knight Lowe Professor, Division of Clinical Immunology and Rheumatology, Vice Chair, Department of Medicine, University of Alabama Birmingham, Birmingham, Alabama, USA

C. MICHAEL SAMSON, MD, MBA
Department of Ophthalmology, Manhattan Eye, Ear, and Throat Hospital, Zucker School of Medicine at Hofstra/Northwell, Hempstead, New York, USA

SEBASTIAN E. SATTUI, MD
Division of Rheumatology, Department of Medicine, Hospital for Special Surgery, New York, New York, USA

MONICA SCHWARTZMAN, MD
Rheumatology Fellow, Department of Medicine, Division of Rheumatology, The Hospital for Special Surgery, New York, New York, USA

SERGIO SCHWARTZMAN, MD
Franchellie M. Cadwell Associate Professor of Medicine, Hospital for Special Surgery, New York Presbyterian Hospital, Weill Medical College of Cornell University, New York, New York, USA

PAIGE N. SCUDDER, MLIS
Biomedical Libraries, Dartmouth College, Hanover, New Hampshire, USA

JOSEF S. SMOLEN, MD
Division of Rheumatology, Department of Internal Medicine 3, Medical University Vienna, Austria

ROBERT F. SPIERA, MD
Division of Rheumatology, Department of Medicine; Professor, Department of Clinical Medicine, Weill Cornell Medical College, Director, Scleroderma, Vasculitis & Myositis Center, Hospital for Special Surgery, New York, New York, USA

JULIA SPIERINGS, MD
Rheumatologist, Department of Rheumatology and Clinical Immunology, University Medical Center Utrecht, Utrecht, the Netherlands

JACOB M. VAN LAAR, MD, PhD
Professor, Head, Department of Rheumatology and Clinical Immunology, University Medical Center Utrecht, Utrecht, the Netherlands

WEIYU YE, BA, MB BChir
Academic Foundation Trainee, Oxford University Clinical Academic Graduate School, University of Oxford, John Radcliffe Hospital (Main Hospital), Oxford, United Kingdom

Contents

Foreword: Controversies in Rheumatology xiii

Michael H. Weisman

Preface: Controversies in Rheumatology xv

Jonathan Kay and Sergio Schwartzman

Does Triple Conventional Synthetic Disease-Modifying Antirheumatic Drug Therapy Improve upon Methotrexate as the Initial Treatment of Choice for a Rheumatoid Arthritis Patient? 315

Daniel Aletaha and Josef S. Smolen

Although many treatment options exist for the initial management of rheumatoid arthritis, there has long been discussion about whether initial treatment should be with methotrexate (MTX) as monotherapy or in combination with other conventional synthetic disease-modifying antirheumatic drugs (csDMARDs). Although studies initially showed additional benefit from combining MTX with other csDMARDs, this benefit disappears when glucocorticoids are added to MTX, a strategy recommended in current guidelines as a short-term bridging approach until MTX therapy exhibits its full efficacy. Also concomitant use of glucocorticoids, with MTX may not be inferior to combination therapy of MTX with TNF-inhibitors.

Should Methotrexate Have Any Place in the Treatment of Psoriatic Arthritis? 325

Weiyu Ye and Laura C. Coates

Methotrexate (MTX) is widely used in the treatment of psoriatic arthritis (PsA), despite the evidence base for this being limited. This narrative review summarizes the evidence to date of using MTX within different domains of psoriatic disease, including peripheral arthritis, axial disease, dactylitis, enthesitis, psoriasis, and nail disease. We also explore the role of MTX in combination therapy with tumor necrosis factor inhibitors, in addition to its safety and tolerability, to answer the question: should methotrexate have any place in the treatment of psoriatic arthritis?

Is There a Role for MRI to Establish Treatment Indications and Effectively Monitor Response in Patients with Axial Spondyloarthritis? 341

Monica Schwartzman and Walter P. Maksymowych

MRI has an important role in the assessment of axial spondyloarthritis (axSpA), particularly early in the disease course, before radiographic damage is apparent. For this reason, MRI was incorporated into the 2009 ASAS/OMERACT classification criteria for spondyloarthritis. However, there are current controversies regarding its use. Important questions include whether the spine should be used in the routine diagnosis and classification of axSpA, whether MRI should replace radiographs as the imaging modality of choice in axSpA, and whether MRI findings in axSpA have prognostic significance.

Are the Current Recommendations for Chloroquine and Hydroxychloroquine Screening Appropriate? 359

Sergio Schwartzman and C. Michael Samson

Hydroxychloroquine and quinacrine are frequently used to treat rheumatic diseases. Ocular toxicity, although infrequent, is one of the potential side effects of antimalarial therapies. Current recommendations are unifocal in being developed by only ophthalmologists who do not treat patients for their rheumatic diseases. The data used to create the recommendations are meager and retrospective. Comanagement of patients with rheumatic disease who are exposed to antimalarial therapies requires a greater interaction between ophthalmologists and rheumatologists.

Should Generalized Immunosuppression or Targeted Organ Treatment be the Best Principle for Overall Management of Systemic Lupus Erythematosus? 369

Nancy Olsen

Systemic lupus erythematosus (SLE) is a systemic autoimmune disease, and standard therapy algorithms include the use of agents with generalized immunosuppressive effects. The outcomes for SLE patients have been markedly improved by this approach. However, the concept that involved organs might be targeted for treatment in an individual patient has potential to provide further benefits, offering enhanced efficacy and fewer off-target effects. This review considers how two of the most commonly involved organ systems in SLE, skin and kidney, might be targets for new therapeutic approaches based on knowledge of underlying mechanisms of disease.

Treatment of Antineutrophil Cytoplasmic Antibody-Associated Vasculitis: Is There Still a Role for Cyclophosphamide? 379

Sebastian E. Sattui and Robert F. Spiera

Antineutrophil cytoplasmic antibody (ANCA)-associated vasculitis (AAV) is a group of systemic necrotizing vasculitides that includes granulomatosis with polyangiitis, microscopic polyangiitis, and eosinophilic granulomatosis with polyangiitis. Treatment of these conditions has improved during the past 2 decades with better understanding of these conditions and availability of newer agents. Cyclophosphamide (CYC) was the first drug demonstrated to afford successful treatment and improvement in AAV. With the emergence of newer agents with more favorable safety profiles, CYC is no longer the cornerstone of management of AAV. This article reviews existing data for treatment and the current role of CYC in the management of AAV.

Is There a Place for Hematopoietic Stem Cell Transplantation in Rheumatology? 399

Julia Spierings and Jacob M. van Laar

In a time where new immunomodulatory therapies are widely available, it seems remarkable that the number of hematopoietic stem cell transplantations (HSCT) performed in rheumatic diseases is still increasing. However, in progressive systemic sclerosis, autologous HSCT is the only treatment with proven survival benefits. In refractory cases of inflammatory arthritis, systemic lupus erythematosus, and several other rare rheumatic conditions, HSCT contributed to better disease control as well. Nevertheless, HSCT is still associated with considerable risks, and a careful balancing of benefits and risks remains paramount.

Should Platelet-Rich Plasma or Stem Cell Therapy Be Used to Treat Osteoarthritis? **417**

Hani Rashid and C. Kent Kwoh

Osteoarthritis is the most common form of arthritis and unfortunately lacks disease-modifying treatments. This has led to a growing demand for more effective nonoperative treatment options. Platelet-rich plasma and mesenchymal stem cell therapy offer the potential to modify the natural course of knee osteoarthritis using cell-based technology. Because of the lack of high-quality evidence and the large degree of heterogeneity, in terms of study designs and measured outcomes, the use of platelet-rich plasma or mesenchymal stem cell therapy to treat knee osteoarthritis cannot be recommended at this time.

Intra-articular Hyaluronan Therapy for Symptomatic Knee Osteoarthritis **439**

Carrie Richardson, Anna Plaas, and Joel A. Block

Intra-articular hyaluronan therapy (IAHA) is a common but controversial nonsurgical treatment of symptomatic knee osteoarthritis. The overall treatment effect of IAHA for osteoarthritis pain is substantial, but the majority of this benefit is mediated by the placebo effect. Despite the large overall benefit of IAHA when the effect of the hyaluronan is combined with the placebo effect, there is only a small benefit of questionable clinical significance of IAHA compared with intra-articular placebo. Compared with intra-articular corticosteroids, however, IAHA most likely is comparable for long-term pain relief and possibly slightly inferior for short-term pain relief.

Vascular Consequences of Hyperuricemia and Hypouricemia **453**

Daniel Albert, Paige N. Scudder, Pamela Bagley, and Kenneth G. Saag

There are more than 10,000 articles in the literature published since 1999 that appear in a search of hyperuricemia and hypouricemia for vascular events. Systematic reviews were reviewed for this time frame, numbering approximately 300 articles in addition to more than 400 reports of randomized clinical trials published since 2017. In summary, the epidemiologic associations of hyperuricemia and hypouricemia with vascular disease are confounded by comorbid conditions. The interventional data are suggestive of a relationship of gout and vascular disease and to a lesser extent hyperuricemia and hypertension; however, more interventional studies are necessary to confirm these relationships.

Are There Benefits and Risks to Biosimilars from a Patient Perspective? **465**

Jonathan Kay

Biosimilars are copies of biologic medications, which no longer are protected by patent, that are intended to be marketed at lower prices than their reference products to increase patient access to treatment. Because a biosimilar must have equivalent pharmacokinetic parameters and efficacy and comparable safety and immunogenicity with its reference

product, the only significant difference between the two should be cost. Lower-priced biosimilars are intended to introduce market competition. The availability of biosimilars should yield savings for the health care system and improve treatment outcomes by expanding patient access to effective medications. However, patients should partake of these cost savings.

RHEUMATIC DISEASE CLINICS OF NORTH AMERICA

FORTHCOMING ISSUES

November 2019
Treat to Target in Rheumatic Diseases: Rationale and Results
Daniel Aletaha, *Editor*

February 2020
Education and Professional Development in Rheumatology
James Katz and Karina Torralba, *Editors*

May 2020
Spondyloarthritis: The Changing Landscape Today
Xenofon Baraliakos and Michael Weisman, *Editors*

RECENT ISSUES

May 2019
Technology and Big Data in Rheumatology
Jeffrey R. Curtis, Kaleb Michaud, and Kevin Winthrop, *Editors*

February 2019
Best Practices and Challenges to the Practice of Rheumatology
Daniel J. Wallace and Swamy Venuturupalli, *Editors*

November 2018
Renal Involvement in Rheumatic Diseases
Andrew Bomback and Meghan E. Sise, *Editors*

Foreword
Controversies in Rheumatology

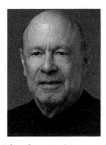

Michael H. Weisman, MD
Consulting Editor

Kay and Schwartzman have submitted to the reader a very thoughtful assessment of some of the most important controversies facing the rheumatologist clinician today, especially regarding therapeutic choices in commonly encountered situations. Their choices of topics and experts are timely, as follows.

Drs Aletaha and Smolen, arguing from a world of clinical and trial experience, reexamine the role of methotrexate with or without a combination of other conventional disease-modifying antirheumatic drugs (DMARDs) in the initial management of a rheumatoid arthritis patient. They conclude that both trial experiences and old-fashioned clinical judgment do not justify favoring a combination of conventional DMARDs over the current guidelines approach consisting of methotrexate plus a short-term use of oral corticosteroids as an initial step before advancing to a biologic drug if necessary. Drs Albert, Scudder, Bagley, and Saag address the controversy surrounding the putative and clearly clinically important associations between hyperuricemia and hypouricemia and vascular events; they note that the epidemiologic and clinical trial data are too confounded by comorbid conditions and possible indirect effects to draw solid conclusions. Jon Kay, an expert in this area, tells us that the major advance for biosimilars in our specialty would be to provide lower-priced alternatives to what we have currently and yield a net cost-savings for the health care system as well as provide access to an expanded patient population. Drs Spierings and van Laar critically review the current state-of-the-art for hematopoietic stem cell transplantation in rheumatic diseases; they conclude that in progressive systemic sclerosis (where there are few options available) there is sufficient justification for its use. Sattui and Spiera, experts in the world of AAV therapeutic options, address the current and future employment of cyclophosphamide for successful treatment and outcomes in these conditions. They conclude that although cyclophosphamide is no longer the cornerstone of treatment, it does have a role for remission-induction in the most

Rheum Dis Clin N Am 45 (2019) xiii–xiv
https://doi.org/10.1016/j.rdc.2019.05.001

severely ill patients, specifically those that have a rapid decline in renal function or those with severe alveolar hemorrhage requiring ventilator support.

Ye and Coates explore the controversial role, if any, for methotrexate (alone, or in combination) in the management of psoriatic arthritis in the biologic era. Schwartzman and Samson examine the current recommendations for screening approaches regarding ocular toxicity for antimalarial agents; they conclude that the current recommendations are one-sided without careful considerations regarding the opinions of rheumatologists who assume, unlike ophthalmologists, the burden of addressing clinical need. They request collaboration between ophthalmologist and rheumatologist specialties to determine a rational approach. Schwartzman and Maksymowych address the evolving role of MRI in spondyloarthritis, the importance of which is quite evident from the controversies concerning its use as a diagnostic or prognostic tool. Does it predict evolution into progressive damage? Is diagnostic specificity as good as we would like considering many similar changes that are seen in healthies? Nancy Olsen examines the main controversy in lupus therapeutics, should generalized immunosuppression (which we now use) give way to targeting cells that cause tissue-specific effects intrinsic to the important involved organs in our patients? Drs Rashid and Kwoh give the reader an important scholarly perspective on the movement of the increasing highly touted use of platelet-rich plasma and mesenchymal stem cell therapies for osteoarthritis. Finally, Drs Richardson, Plaas, and Block provide a balanced view on the widespread use of intraarticular hyaluronan therapy for symptomatic knee osteoarthritis. They feel, after the review of trials and meta-analyses, that the majority of the pain-relieving effect is small and of questionable clinical significance over intraarticular placebo administration.

Michael H. Weisman, MD
David Geffen School of Medicine at UCLA
Cedars-Sinai Medical Center
1545 Calmar Court
Los Angeles, CA 90024, USA

E-mail address:
Michael.Weisman@csh.org

Preface
Controversies in Rheumatology

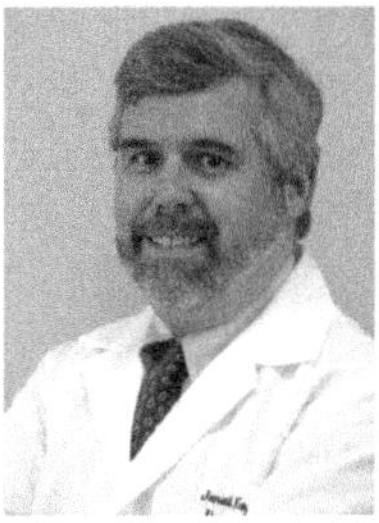
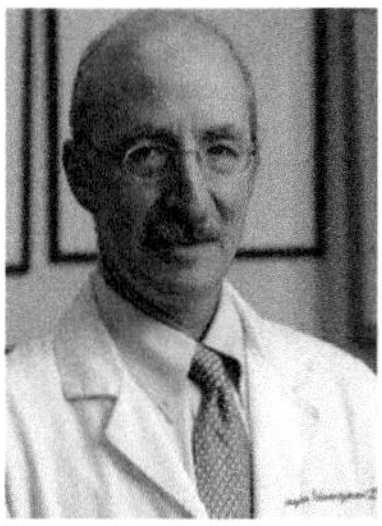

Jonathan Kay, MD Sergio Schwartzman, MD
Editors

Rheumatology is a relatively young subspecialty, first recognized in 1925 when the International Committee on Rheumatism was founded by Jan van Breeman at the first meeting of the International Society of Medical Hydrology in Paris.[1] As such, research into the pathophysiology, clinical presentation, and treatment of the rheumatic diseases and the development of classification criteria for individual conditions continues to advance, as our subspecialty is poised to enter its second century.

There are a very small number of absolute facts in rheumatology. The few incontrovertible truths include such observations as that negatively birefringent crystals are present in synovial fluid of patients with gout and that the presence of IgG anti-cyclic citrullinated peptide antibodies correlates with the development of rheumatoid arthritis. However, even those statements can be debated. It has been said that, if 2 rheumatologists evaluate the same patient, they may come up with at least 3 different opinions. Thus, as with Talmudic scholars, controversy is commonplace among rheumatologists.

In this issue, we have identified only a few of the current "controversies" in rheumatology. Perhaps, a more apropos term might have been "discussions," since we anticipate that ongoing research will soon generate new data that will help to resolve the questions proposed in each of the 11 articles in this issue. Also, new questions and controversies are certain to arise, any of which would be appropriate to include in a future issue bearing the same title as this one.

We hope that the reader will enjoy both our choice of topics and the erudite discussions provided by each of the contributors. Most importantly, we expect that open

Rheum Dis Clin N Am 45 (2019) xv–xvi
https://doi.org/10.1016/j.rdc.2019.05.002
0889-857X/19/© 2019 Published by Elsevier Inc.
rheumatic.theclinics.com

discussion of these and other controversial topics will continue to stimulate systematic investigation, which is an attribute that defines our subspecialty.

Jonathan Kay, MD
UMass Memorial Medical Center
University of Massachusetts Medical School
119 Belmont Street
Worcester, MA 01605, USA

Sergio Schwartzman, MD
Hospital for Special Surgery
New York Presbyterian Hospital
Weill Medical College of Cornell University
535 East 70th Street, 8th Floor
New York, NY 10021, USA

E-mail addresses:
jonathan.kay@umassmemorial.org (J. Kay)
ssrheum@gmail.com (S. Schwartzman)

REFERENCE

1. Stecher RM. The American Rheumatism Association—its origins, development and maturity. Arthritis Rheum 1958;1(1):4–19.

Does Triple Conventional Synthetic Disease-Modifying Antirheumatic Drug Therapy Improve upon Methotrexate as the Initial Treatment of Choice for a Rheumatoid Arthritis Patient?

Daniel Aletaha, MD*, Josef S. Smolen, MD

KEYWORDS

- Methotrexate monotherapy • Triple therapy • Combination therapy
- Rheumatoid arthritis • Biological DMARDs

KEY POINTS

- In the presence of glucocorticoids, no efficacy differences exist between methotrexate monotherapy and combination conventional synthetic DMARD (csDMARD) therapy
- Combination csDMARD therapy is similarly effective, but less safe, in rheumatoid arthritis in the presence of glucocorticoids.
- A step-up approach from initial MTX monotherapy to triple csDMARD therapy is unlikely to result in a clinically relevant response in most patients.

INTRODUCTION: SETTING THE SCENE

The treatment of rheumatoid arthritis (RA) focuses on reversing signs and symptoms, normalizing physical function and quality of life, and preventing the development or progression of joint damage.[1] Signs and symptoms, such as joint swelling,

---

Disclosure Statement: D. Aletaha: Research grants: Abbvie, Novartis, Roche; Speakers bureau/ Consultancy: Abbvie, Amgen, Celgene, Lilly, Medac, Merck, Novartis, Pfizer, Roche, Sandoz, Sanofi/Genzyme. J.S. Smolen: Research grants: AbbVie, BMS, Lilly, MSD, Novartis, Pfizer, and Roche; Speakers bureau/Consultancy: Abbvie, Astra-Zeneca, BMS, Boehringer Ingelheim, Celgene, Celltrion, Gilead, ILTOO, Janssen, Lilly, Novartis-Sandoz, Pfizer, Roche, Samsung, Sanofi, and UCB.
Division of Rheumatology, Department of Internal Medicine 3, Medical University Vienna, Spitalgasse 23, 1090 Vienna, Austria
* Corresponding author.
E-mail address: daniel.aletaha@meduniwien.ac.at

Rheum Dis Clin N Am 45 (2019) 315–324
https://doi.org/10.1016/j.rdc.2019.04.002
rheumatic.theclinics.com

tenderness, pain, and stiffness, are primarily a consequence of the inflammatory processes that occur in the synovial membrane (typically referred to as "synovitis"). Studies of the mechanisms responsible for joint damage reveal that cartilage destruction results from the direct action of metalloproteinases secreted by synovial fibroblasts and macrophages, as well as from the activation of chondrocytes by proinflammatory cytokines. At the same time, it seems that juxta-articular subchondral bone destruction is due to the stimulation and resorptive actions of osteoclasts that are mediated by the effects of activated synovial cells and proinflammatory cytokines on osteoclast precursors.[2,3] Joint damage generally is regarded as being irreversible, with the exception of some small, early changes. Finally, physical disability is a consequence of both disease activity (reflected by pain and stiffness) and joint damage; these 2 components have different consequences, because disease activity is reversible whereas joint damage is not.[4,5] These characteristics of the "RA triad" are depicted schematically in **Fig. 1**. In addition to joint damage, disability is also brought about by comorbidities,[6] such as cardiovascular disease, which are a further consequence of the preceding inflammatory events.[7,8]

Thus, since inflammation drives all aspects of RA that are detrimental to patients, either directly through signs and symptoms or indirectly through damage, disability, and comorbidities, the principal target of RA treatment is the attainment of remission or, when applying the treat-to-target (T2T) approach,[9] at least reducing inflammation to the level of a low state of disease activity. Hence, every therapeutic approach in RA has to be viewed primarily through the "T2T prism" to define a therapeutic target that is applicable to all patients.

THERAPIES AVAILABLE TO TREAT RHEUMATOID ARTHRITIS

Never before have there been as many medications available to treat patients with RA. In addition to several conventional synthetic disease-modifying antirheumatic drugs (csDMARDs), such as methotrexate (MTX), sulfasalazine (SSZ), leflunomide, hydroxychloroquine (HCQ), and chloroquine, a large number of biological DMARDs (bDMARDs) are available, including several tumor necrosis factor (TNF) inhibitors, interleukin-6 (IL-6) receptor blockers, abatacept, and rituximab. Also, the Janus kinase

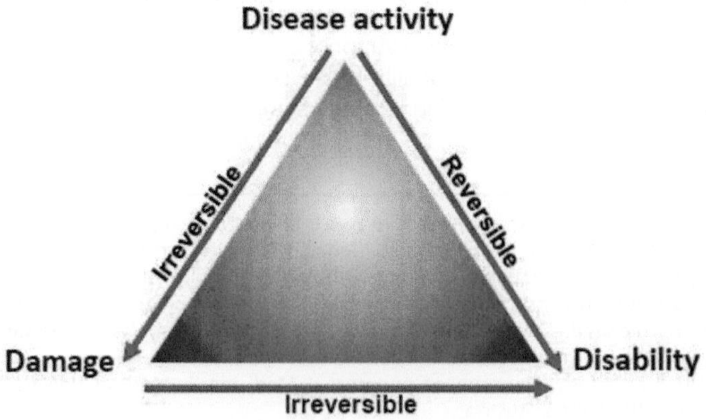

Fig. 1. Relationship between disease activity, damage, and disability. (*Adapted from* Smolen JS, Schöls M, Braun J, et al. Treating axial spondyloarthritis and peripheral spondyloarthritis, especially psoriatic arthritis, to target: 2017 update of recommendations by an international task force. Ann Rheum Dis 2018;77(1):3–17. https://doi.org/10.1136/annrheumdis-2017-211734. Epub 2017 Jul 6; with permission.)

(Jak) inhibitors, tofacitinib and baricitinib, are now available as targeted synthetic DMARDs (tsDMARDs) that inhibit signaling through a variety of cytokine receptors to reduce inflammation and its consequences.[10] In addition, glucocorticoids (GCs) exert strong anti-inflammatory effects, especially as bridging therapy when added upon initiating csDMARD treatment.[11]

Several bDMARDs and tsDMARDs exhibit better efficacy when used in combination with a csDMARD, especially MTX, than when used as monotherapy.[12–16] It also has been postulated that combinations of csDMARDs may be more effective than when individual csDMARDs are administered as monotherapy, particularly for the triple csDMARD therapy regimen of MTX, SSZ, and HCQ.[17] Likewise, treatment with MTX in combination with a GC results in better outcomes than treatment with MTX alone[18,19] and outcomes similar to those for the combination of MTX with an anti-TNF agent.[20] It is in the context of these data, which have been derived over the last decade, that we address the current status of triple csDMARD therapy when compared with treatment with MTX alone or with MTX in combination with other medications, such as bDMARDs.

TRIPLE CONVENTIONAL SYNTHETIC DISEASE-MODIFYING ANTIRHEUMATIC DRUG THERAPY IN COMPARISON WITH METHOTREXATE MONOTHERAPY

Treatment with the triple csDMARD therapy regimen, consisting of the combination of MTX, SSZ, and HCQ, was suggested to be superior to treatment with MTX alone or with the combination of SSZ and HCQ in a double-blind randomized clinical trial published in 1996.[17] This was a small trial that enrolled only 31 to 36 RA patients with disease of about 10-year duration into each of the 3 arms. SSZ was dosed at only 1000 mg/d, which today would be considered to be an ineffective dose for SSZ monotherapy. Oral MTX was started at 7.5 mg weekly and the dose was increased to 12.5 mg weekly at month 3 and to 17.5 mg weekly at month 6, a dose-escalation schedule that now would be regarded as too slow because the dose of MTX typically is increased to between 20 mg and 25 mg within 8 weeks.[21] The primary end point was a 50% improvement in the modified Paulus criteria, which were the predecessor of the American College of Rheumatology (ACR) improvement criteria; thus, this end point corresponds more or less to an ACR_{50} (ie, 50% improvement) response. At month 9, patients who did not achieve a 50% improvement in the modified Paulus criteria were withdrawn from the study. At 24 months, 77% of the patients who had received triple csDMARD therapy showed a 50% improvement in the modified Paulus criteria, compared with 33% of the patients who had been treated with MTX alone. This response rate observed with MTX monotherapy is consistent with that which was experienced in the 1990s by patients with early RA (<3 years' duration) who were treated with MTX.[22] However, no other clinical trial of any other drug regimen has ever yielded anything near a 50% clinical response rate of 77%. Thus, we interpret these results as a "play of chance" owing to the small number of subjects enrolled in each arm of the study. As we have pointed out previously, the triple csDMARD therapy arm had fewer subjects than the other 2 arms, despite randomization, and had a lower mean baseline erythrocyte sedimentation rate and 10% to 15% lower mean tender and swollen joint counts than those of the other 2 arms.[23]

The Fin-RACo trial compared the combination of triple csDMARD therapy with prednisone with treatment of RA with SSZ alone.[24] In this study, 97 patients were treated the combination of MTX, SSZ, HCQ, and prednisolone and 98 patients received SSZ alone or with prednisolone. The primary end point was induction of remission, as defined according to the 1981 American Rheumatism Association (now the ACR) preliminary criteria for clinical remission in RA by Pinals and colleagues,[25] excluding fatigue and drug withdrawal. At 1 year, this end point was achieved by 24 of the 97 patients who were treated with combination therapy and by 11 of the 98 patients who were treated initially with SSZ monotherapy ($P = .011$). In a previous review[23] we pointed out that (1) this study was open-label, (2) there were imbalances between groups, including higher joint damage and swollen and tender joint counts in the monotherapy group, and (3) there were differences in the approach to initiating GC treatment (from the start in the combination therapy group and, usually, at some later time point in the SSZ monotherapy group), which may have contributed to the more favorable outcomes observed in the group treated with combination therapy.

That this imbalance in GC use, indeed, was most likely the reason for the differential outcomes in Fin-RACo was ultimately confirmed in 2 subsequent trials in which combination csDMARD therapy plus GC were compared with the combination of MTX alone with GC. In the tREACH trial, 97 patients received MTX monotherapy plus oral GCs, 93 patients received triple csDMARD therapy plus oral GCs, and 91 patients received triple csDMARD therapy plus intramuscular GCs.[26] Although there was a trend in favor of triple csDMARD therapy, the differences between treatment arms in clinical, functional, and radiographic outcome measures were not statistically significant. Moreover, there were fewer adverse events and treatment discontinuations in the MTX monotherapy plus GC arm (**Fig. 2**).[26] These findings were confirmed in the CareRA trial, which compared treatment of RA with MTX plus prednisone 30 mg (n = 98), the combination of MTX with SSZ plus prednisone 60 mg (n = 98), and the combination of MTX with leflunomide plus prednisone 30 mg. In this study there were no clinical or functional differences between treatment groups; however, the incidence of adverse events was significantly lower in the MTX monotherapy plus GC arm.[27] A systematic literature review that was performed to inform the European League Against Rheumatism (EULAR) RA management recommendations also did not find sufficient evidence to support the superiority of combination csDMARD therapy to treatment with a single csDMARD plus GCs.[28] In fact, these recommendations now clearly advocate the concomitant short-term use of GCs when initiating csDMARD treatment.[29]

TRIPLE CONVENTIONAL SYNTHETIC DISEASE-MODIFYING ANTIRHEUMATIC DRUG THERAPY IN COMPARISON WITH BIOLOGICAL DISEASE-MODIFYING ANTIRHEUMATIC DRUG THERAPY

As mentioned earlier, treatment with csDMARDs in combination with GCs results in better clinical, functional, and structural outcomes than with csDMARD therapy alone. Alternatively, treatment with the combination of bDMARDs and csDMARDs also results in better outcomes than does initiation of treatment with MTX alone.[22,30–32] Treatment with the tsDMARD Jak inhibitors yields similar results with or without concomitant csDMARDs.[33,34] However, whereas large registration trials of novel medications traditionally have assessed the efficacy of a new treatment in patients already taking MTX (or, in some patients, in addition to stable background GCs), new drugs were never assessed in comparison with the combination of MTX plus GC during the development process. This assessment, however, ultimately was carried out in investigator-initiated trials in MTX-naïve patients and revealed, surprisingly, that treatment with the combination of a bDMARD plus MTX was not superior to treatment with MTX plus GC by any outcome measure, either clinical, functional, or structural.[20,35] These findings were pivotal when EULAR formulated the recommendation to treat early RA with the combination of MTX plus GC, rather than with a bDMARD or a tsDMARD.[29]

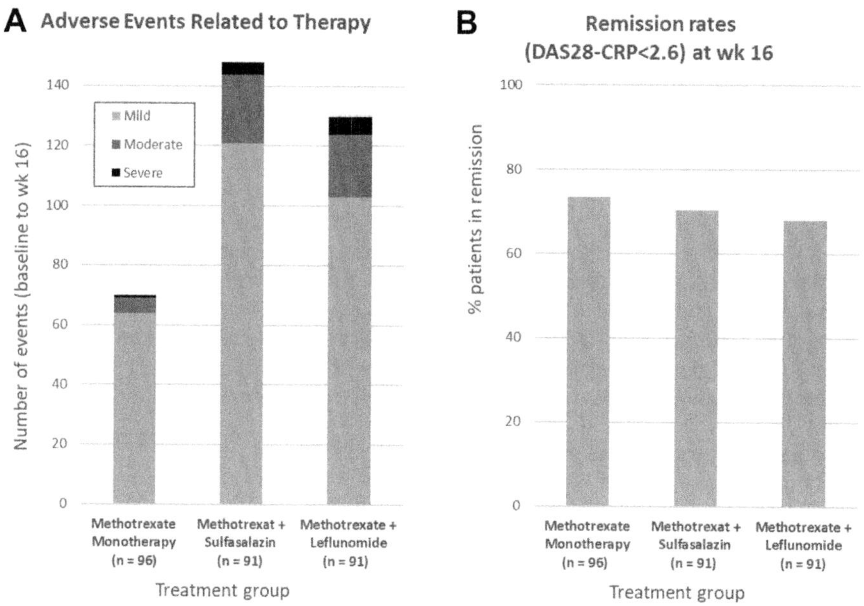

Fig. 2. Adverse events and their severity (*A*) and efficacy (*B*) from the CareRA trial[27] comparing methotrexate monotherapy with the combination of methotrexate with either sulfasalazine or leflunomide. Subjects in all treatment arms received glucocorticoids. Please take into consideration that a DAS28 score of less than 2.6 overrates remission because of underrating swollen joint counts as well as overrating tender joint counts and acute phase reactants. Thus, patients may exhibit significant residual disease activity and radiographic progression while in DAS28 "remission."[46,47] However, in this study all treatment arms received glucocorticoids. Therefore, although this cut point reflects low disease activity rather than remission,[48] differences in response rates are not to be expected, in contrast to comparisons of agents that interfere with IL-6 pathways with other drugs.[49,50] (*Data from* de Jong PH, Hazes JM, Han HK, Huisman M, van ZD, van der Lubbe PA, et al. Randomised comparison of initial triple DMARD therapy with methotrexate monotherapy in combination with low-dose glucocorticoid bridging therapy; 1-year data of the tREACH trial. Ann Rheum Dis 2014; 73(7):1331–1339.)

Results of recent trials have suggested that treatment of RA with triple csDMARD therapy is not inferior to the combination of a bDMARD with MTX.[36,37] In the RACAT trial, patients who had responded inadequately to MTX were randomized either to step up to triple csDMARD therapy, by adding SSZ and HCQ, or to the addition of a biological DMARD, etanercept. In this noninferiority study, the primary end point was improvement in the 28-joint disease activity score (DAS28) at 48 weeks. However, because enrollment was unexpectedly slow, the study did not reach its targeted sample size and the primary end point was changed during the course of the study. Although the study met its revised primary end point, only 5% of patients receiving triple csDMARD therapy achieved an ACR_{70} response, in contrast to 16% of patients receiving etanercept and MTX. As ACR_{70} responses are a surrogate of low disease activity, which is the target of the T2T strategy, this was both a clinically and statistically significant difference favoring the bDMARD-treated group. However, even the difference in the proportions of ACR_{50} responders almost reached statistical significance in favor of bDMARD plus MTX therapy. This was recently confirmed by meta-analyses.[38,39] For these reasons, the conclusion of the RACAT trial that triple csDMARD therapy is noninferior to bDMARD plus MTX treatment is inaccurate. Several publications have appeared subsequently which demonstrate that triple csDMARD therapy is poorly tolerated,[40,41] providing another reason to avoid using this treatment.

The cost of bDMARDs is much greater than that of combination csDMARD therapy. However, in today's world cost is a moving target, and: (1) if the treatment algorithm recommended by EULAR is followed, using MTX plus GC as initial therapy,[29] more than 50% of patients will attain the treatment target of low disease activity or remission; (2) with the availability of biosimilars, the cost of bDMARDs has been reduced by up to 70%[42]; and (3) as duration of disease activity before initiation of effective therapy contributes importantly to refractoriness of RA,[43,44] there is no reason to initiate a treatment with little chance of being highly effective and for which there is a high probability of developing adverse events.

SUMMARY AND RECOMMENDATIONS

Recent clinical trials have shown that MTX plus short-term GC is similarly effective to triple csDMARD therapy plus GC. Thus, there is no place for triple csDMARD therapy at the beginning of the treatment algorithm for RA, especially as adverse events occur more frequently with this combination than with MTX monotherapy. When a patient with RA fails to achieve remission or low disease activity on MTX monotherapy, there is little further benefit to adding other csDMARDs.[45] This clinical observation was confirmed in the RACAT trial, in which ACR_{70} responses were achieved by only 5% of patients who had responded inadequately to MTX when they were advanced to triple csDMARD therapy.[37] However, because no placebo group was included in this study, it is not known whether triple csDMARD therapy would have been more effective than placebo for this outcome measure. Also, progression of joint damage was significantly higher in patients treated with triple csDMARD therapy than with the addition of a TNF inhibitor to MTX. Consequently, when MTX therapy has failed, the use of triple csDMARD therapy should be limited to situations in which both bDMARDs and tsDMARDs are contraindicated.

In summary, the initial treatment of choice for RA is MTX with a short-term GC. No clinical trial has shown the efficacy and safety of this therapy to be surpassed by any other regimen. When this treatment fails, a bDMARD or tsDMARD should be added to MTX as the next step of choice. Triple csDMARD therapy has little, if any, place at this point in the therapeutic algorithm. Data accumulated over the past decade confirm the validity of the 2016 EULAR RA management recommendations,[29] which advocate this approach.

REFERENCES

1. Aletaha D, Smolen JS. Diagnosis and management of rheumatoid arthritis: a review. JAMA 2018;320(13):1360–72.
2. Redlich K, Smolen JS. Inflammatory bone loss: pathogenesis and therapeutic intervention. Nat Rev Drug Discov 2012;11(3):234–50.
3. Puchner A, Saferding V, Bonelli M, et al. Non-classical monocytes as mediators of tissue destruction in arthritis. Ann Rheum Dis 2018;77(10):1490–7.
4. Aletaha D, Smolen J, Ward MM. Measuring function in rheumatoid arthritis: identifying reversible and irreversible components. Arthritis Rheum 2006;54:2784–92.

5. Smolen JS, Aletaha D, Grisar JC, et al. Estimation of a numerical value for joint damage-related physical disability in rheumatoid arthritis clinical trials. Ann Rheum Dis 2010;69(6):1058–64.
6. Radner H, Smolen JS, Aletaha D. Impact of comorbidity on physical function in patients with rheumatoid arthritis. Ann Rheum Dis 2010;69(3):536–41.
7. Innala L, Moller B, Ljung L, et al. Cardiovascular events in early RA are a result of inflammatory burden and traditional risk factors: a five year prospective study. Arthritis Res Ther 2011;13(4):R131.
8. Grisar J, Aletaha D, Steiner CW, et al. Depletion of endothelial progenitor cells in the peripheral blood of patients with rheumatoid arthritis. Circulation 2005;111: 204–11.
9. Smolen JS, Breedveld FC, Burmester GR, et al. Treating rheumatoid arthritis to target: 2014 update of the recommendations of an international task force. Ann Rheum Dis 2016;75(1):3–15.
10. Smolen JS, Aletaha D, Barton A, et al. Rheumatoid arthritis. Nat Rev Dis Primers 2018;4:18001.
11. Hoes JN, Jacobs JW, Boers M, et al. EULAR evidence-based recommendations on the management of systemic glucocorticoid therapy in rheumatic diseases. Ann Rheum Dis 2007;66(12):1560–7.
12. Maini RN, Breedveld FC, Kalden JR, et al. Therapeutic efficacy of multiple intravenous infusions of anti-tumor necrosis factor alpha monoclonal antibody combined with low-dose weekly methotrexate in rheumatoid arthritis. Arthritis Rheum 1998;41(9):1552–63.
13. Kaneko Y, Atsumi T, Tanaka Y, et al. Comparison of adding tocilizumab to methotrexate with switching to tocilizumab in patients with rheumatoid arthritis with inadequate response to methotrexate: 52-week results from a prospective, randomised, controlled study (SURPRISE study). Ann Rheum Dis 2016;75(11): 1917–23.
14. Edwards JC, Szczepanski L, Szechinski J, et al. Efficacy of B-cell-targeted therapy with rituximab in patients with rheumatoid arthritis. N Engl J Med 2004;350: 2572–81.
15. Fleischmann R, Schiff M, van der Heijde D, et al. Baricitinib, methotrexate, or combination in patients with rheumatoid arthritis and no or limited prior disease-modifying antirheumatic drug treatment. Arthritis Rheumatol 2017; 69(3):506–17.
16. Fleischmann R, Mysler E, Hall S, et al. Efficacy and safety of tofacitinib monotherapy, tofacitinib with methotrexate, and adalimumab with methotrexate in patients with rheumatoid arthritis (ORAL Strategy): a phase 3b/4, double-blind, head-to-head, randomised controlled trial. Lancet 2017;390:457–68.
17. O'Dell J. Treatment of rheumatoid arthritis with methotrexate alone, sulfasalazine and hydroxychloroquine, or a combination of all three medications. N Engl J Med 1996;334:1287–91.
18. Svensson B, Boonen A, Albertsson K, et al. Low-dose prednisolone in addition to the initial disease-modifying antirheumatic drug in patients with early active rheumatoid arthritis reduces joint destruction and increases the remission rate: a two-year randomized trial. Arthritis Rheum 2005;52:3360–70.
19. Wassenberg S, Rau R, Steinfeld P, et al. Very low-dose prednisolone in early rheumatoid arthritis retards radiographic progression over two years: a multicenter, double-blind, placebo-controlled trial. Arthritis Rheum 2005;52: 3371–80.

20. Nam JL, Villeneuve E, Hensor EM, et al. Remission induction comparing infliximab and high-dose intravenous steroid, followed by treat-to-target: a double-blind, randomised, controlled trial in new-onset, treatment-naive, rheumatoid arthritis (the IDEA study). Ann Rheum Dis 2014;73(1):75–85.
21. Emery P, Bingham CO III, Burmester GR, et al. Certolizumab pegol in combination with dose-optimised methotrexate in DMARD-naive patients with early, active rheumatoid arthritis with poor prognostic factors: 1-year results from C-EARLY, a randomised, double-blind, placebo-controlled phase III study. Ann Rheum Dis 2017;76:96–104.
22. St Clair EW, van der Heijde DM, Smolen JS, et al. Combination of infliximab and methotrexate therapy for early rheumatoid arthritis: a randomized, controlled trial. Arthritis Rheum 2004;50:3432–43.
23. Smolen JS, Aletaha D, Keystone E. Superior efficacy of combination therapy for rheumatoid arthritis. fact or fiction? Arthritis Rheum 2005;52:2975–83.
24. Mottonen T, Hannonen P, Leirisalo-Repo M, et al. Comparison of combination therapy with single-drug therapy in early rheumatoid arthritis: a randomised trial. FIN-RACo trial group. Lancet 1999;353(9164):1568–73.
25. Pinals RS, Masi AT, Larsen RA. Preliminary criteria for clinical remission in rheumatoid arthritis. Arthritis Rheum 1981;24(1308):1315.
26. de Jong PH, Hazes JM, Han HK, et al. Randomised comparison of initial triple DMARD therapy with methotrexate monotherapy in combination with low-dose glucocorticoid bridging therapy; 1-year data of the tREACH trial. Ann Rheum Dis 2014;73(7):1331–9.
27. Verschueren P, De CD, Corluy L, et al. Methotrexate in combination with other DMARDs is not superior to methotrexate alone for remission induction with moderate-to-high-dose glucocorticoid bridging in early rheumatoid arthritis after 16 weeks of treatment: the CareRA trial. Ann Rheum Dis 2015;74(1):27–34.
28. Chatzidionysiou K, Emamikia S, Nam J, et al. Efficacy of glucocorticoids, conventional and targeted synthetic disease-modifying antirheumatic drugs: a systematic literature review informing the 2016 update of the EULAR recommendations for the management of rheumatoid arthritis. Ann Rheum Dis 2017;76(6):1102–7.
29. Smolen JS, Landewe R, Bijlsma J, et al. EULAR recommendations for the management of rheumatoid arthritis with synthetic and biological disease-modifying antirheumatic drugs: 2016 update. Ann Rheum Dis 2017;76:960–77.
30. Westhovens R, Robles M, Ximenes AC, et al. Clinical efficacy and safety of abatacept in methotrexate-naive patients with early rheumatoid arthritis and poor prognostic factors. Ann Rheum Dis 2009;68:1870–7.
31. Tak PP, Rigby WF, Rubbert-Roth A, et al. Inhibition of joint damage and improved clinical outcomes with rituximab plus methotrexate in early active rheumatoid arthritis: the IMAGE trial. Ann Rheum Dis 2011;70(1):39–46.
32. Burmester GR, Rigby WF, van Vollenhoven RF, et al. Tocilizumab in early progressive rheumatoid arthritis: FUNCTION, a randomised controlled trial. Ann Rheum Dis 2015;75:1081–91.
33. Fleischmann R, Takeuchi T, Schlichting D, et al. Baricitinib, methotrexate, or baricitinib plus methotrexate in patients with early rheumatoid arthritis who had received limited or no treatment with disease-modifying anti-rheumatic drugs (DMARDs): phase 3 trial results [abstract]. Arthritis Rheum 2015;67(Suppl 10). Abstract 1045. Available at: http://acrabstracts.org/abstract/baricitinib-methotrexate-or-baricitinib-plus-methotrexate-in-patients-with-early-rheumatoid-arthritis-who-had-received-limited-or-no-treatment-with-disease-modifying-anti-rheumatic-drugs-dmards-p/. Accessed January 4, 2016.

34. Lee EB, Fleischmann R, Hall S, et al. Tofacitinib versus methotrexate in rheumatoid arthritis. N Engl J Med 2014;370(25):2377–86.
35. Heimans L, Wevers-de Boer KV, Visser K, et al. A two-step treatment strategy trial in patients with early arthritis aimed at achieving remission: the IMPROVED study. Ann Rheum Dis 2014;73(7):1356–61.
36. Moreland LW, O'Dell JR, Paulus HE, et al. A randomized comparative effectiveness study of oral triple therapy versus etanercept plus methotrexate in early aggressive rheumatoid arthritis: the treatment of early aggressive rheumatoid arthritis trial. Arthritis Rheum 2012;64(9):2824–35.
37. O'Dell JR, Mikuls TR, Taylor TH, et al. Therapies for active rheumatoid arthritis after methotrexate failure. N Engl J Med 2013;369:307–18.
38. Bae SC, Lee YH. Comparative efficacy and safety of TNF-inhibitor plus methotrexate versus oral triple therapy in patients with active rheumatoid arthritis inadequately responding to methotrexate: a meta-analysis of randomized controlled trials. Int J Clin Pharmacol Ther 2018;56(6):263–9.
39. Fleischmann R, Tongbram V, van VR, et al. Systematic review and network meta-analysis of the efficacy and safety of tumour necrosis factor inhibitor-methotrexate combination therapy versus triple therapy in rheumatoid arthritis. RMD Open 2017;3(1):e000371.
40. Erhardt DP, Cannon GW, Teng CC, et al. Low persistence rates in rheumatoid arthritis patients treated with triple therapy are attributed to adverse drug events associated with sulfasalazine. Arthritis Care Res (Hoboken) 2018. https://doi.org/10.1002/acr.23759.
41. Verschueren P, De CD, Corluy L, et al. Effectiveness of methotrexate with step-down glucocorticoid remission induction (COBRA Slim) versus other intensive treatment strategies for early rheumatoid arthritis in a treat-to-target approach: 1-year results of CareRA, a randomised pragmatic open-label superiority trial. Ann Rheum Dis 2017;76(3):511–20.
42. Kay J, Schoels MM, Dorner T, et al. Consensus-based recommendations for the use of biosimilars to treat rheumatological diseases. Ann Rheum Dis 2018;77(2):165–74.
43. Aletaha D, Strand V, Smolen JS, et al. Treatment-related improvement in physical function varies with duration of rheumatoid arthritis: a pooled analysis of clinical trial results. Ann Rheum Dis 2008;67(2):238–43.
44. Becede M, Alasti F, Gessl I, et al. Risk profiling for a refractory course of rheumatoid arthritis. Semin Arthritis Rheum 2019. https://doi.org/10.1016/j.semarthrit.2019.02.004.
45. Kiely P, Walsh D, Williams R, et al. Outcome in rheumatoid arthritis patients with continued conventional therapy for moderate disease activity—the early RA network (ERAN). Rheumatology (Oxford) 2011;50(5):926–31.
46. Bakker MF, Jacobs JW, Verstappen SM, et al. Tight control in the treatment of rheumatoid arthritis: efficacy and feasibility. Ann Rheum Dis 2007;66(Suppl 3):iii56–60.
47. Aletaha D, Smolen JS. Joint damage in rheumatoid arthritis progresses in remission according to the Disease Activity Score in 28 joints and is driven by residual swollen joints. Arthritis Rheum 2011;63(12):3702–11.
48. Food and Drug Administration. Guidance for industry—rheumatoid arthritis: developing drug products for treatment. Draft gudance 2013. Available at: http://www.fda.gov/downloads/Drugs/GuidanceComplianceRegulatoryInformation/Guidances/UCM354468.pdf. Accessed October 5, 2013.

49. Smolen JS, Aletaha D. Interleukin-6 receptor inhibition with tocilizumab and attainment of disease remission in rheumatoid arthritis: the role of acute-phase reactants. Arthritis Rheum 2011;63(1):43–52.
50. Smolen JS, Aletaha D, Gruben D, et al. Brief report: remission rates with tofacitinib treatment in rheumatoid arthritis: a comparison of various remission criteria. Arthritis Rheumatol 2017;69(4):728–34.

Should Methotrexate Have Any Place in the Treatment of Psoriatic Arthritis?

Weiyu Ye, BA, MB BChir[a], Laura C. Coates, MB ChB, MRCP, PhD[b,*]

KEYWORDS

• Methotrexate • Psoriatic arthritis • Psoriasis • Treatment • Efficacy

KEY POINTS

- Methotrexate (MTX) is commonly used in the management of psoriatic arthritis.
- There is a paucity of high-quality evidence supporting the efficacy of MTX in psoriatic arthritis, as the available data mainly stem from historical trials with small sample sizes and limited study designs.
- MTX may improve joint symptoms in peripheral arthritis; however, it may not halt radiographic progression.
- MTX is effective in treating psoriasis, and may have a beneficial effect in enthesitis, dactylitis, and nail disease.
- There are limited data on how MTX exerts its beneficial effect in PsA; however, this is likely to be through immunomodulation.

INTRODUCTION

Psoriatic arthritis (PsA) is a chronic inflammatory arthropathy with a significant impact on patients' quality of life.[1] Within PsA, there are several different "domains" of

---

Disclosure Statement: W. Ye is an academic foundation trainee. L.C. Coates is funded by a National Institute for Health Research Clinician Scientist award. The research was supported by the National Institute for Health Research (NIHR) Oxford Biomedical Research Centre (BRC). The views expressed are those of the authors and not necessarily those of the NHS, the NIHR, or the Department of Health. W. Ye has no conflict of interest to declare. L.C. Coates has received research funding from Abbvie, Celgene, Lilly, Novartis, and Pfizer. L.C. Coates has received honoraria from Abbvie, Amgen, Celgene, Galapagos, Gilead, Janssen, Lilly, Novartis, Pfizer, Prothena, Sun Pharma, and UCB.

[a] Oxford University Clinical Academic Graduate School, University of Oxford, John Radcliffe Hospital (Main Hospital), Room 3A31, The Cairns Library IT Corridor, Level 3, Oxford OX3 9DU, UK; [b] Nuffield Department of Orthopaedics, Rheumatology and Musculoskeletal Sciences, Botnar Research Centre, Windmill Road, Oxford OX3 7LD, UK

* Corresponding author.

E-mail address: laura.coates@ndorms.ox.ac.uk

Rheum Dis Clin N Am 45 (2019) 325–339

https://doi.org/10.1016/j.rdc.2019.04.007 rheumatic.theclinics.com

disease, including peripheral arthritis, axial disease, dactylitis, enthesitis, and skin/nail disease, which may vary between different individuals.

Current management is increasingly shifting toward a "treat-to-target" approach, aimed at controlling disease activity through early intervention and regular objective assessments of disease activity, with escalation in therapy if disease control is not achieved. This strategy stems from the results of the Tight Control of Psoriatic Arthritis (TICOPA) study,[2] an open-label multicenter randomized controlled trial of 206 patients with early PsA. The authors demonstrated that patients in the tight control group were more likely to achieve an American College of Rheumatology 20% improvement criteria (ACR20) at 48 weeks compared with patients in the standard care group. To replicate these findings in clinical practice, a full assessment of the different disease domains is required for each patient to enable appropriate therapy effective against the relevant domains to be initiated. In addition, it also requires assessment of overall response, for example, through the minimal disease activity (MDA) criteria.[3]

Currently, methotrexate (MTX) is widely used as the initial therapy in the treatment of PsA, despite limited evidence from high-quality randomized controlled trials to support this approach.[4,5] This is likely due to the assumed effectiveness of MTX from studies in rheumatoid arthritis (RA) and psoriasis. It is highly unlikely that any further placebo-controlled trials assessing the effectiveness of MTX in PsA will be conducted in the future. This is because it defies clinical equipoise and would be extremely hard to recruit for, and it is ethically difficult to justify giving placebo to patients with active PsA when multiple effective treatments for PsA exist.

In this narrative review, we summarize the evidence to date of using MTX in PsA for individual disease domains, as well as in combination with biologic therapy. We also explore the tolerability and adverse effects associated with MTX use in PsA, aiming to answer the question: should MTX be used in the treatment of PsA?

EFFICACY OF METHOTREXATE IN DIFFERENT DOMAINS OF PSORIATIC ARTHRITIS

Peripheral Arthritis

MTX is widely used as a conventional synthetic disease-modifying antirheumatic drug (csDMARD) to treat peripheral arthritis in PsA. However, there is conflicting evidence on whether it is efficacious.

The first double-blind randomized controlled trial of MTX versus placebo was published by Black and colleagues[6] in 1964, using a crossover design. High doses of parenteral MTX were used (1–3 mg/kg) in 21 patients with active peripheral PsA. Compared with placebo, MTX resulted in significant improvements in the joint index (comprising of joint motion, tenderness, and swelling), joint range of motion, and erythrocyte sedimentation rate (ESR). There was also a significant reduction in the percentage of skin area affected. However, there was a high incidence of adverse events (AEs), with 1 patient death. This study was the first to demonstrate that high-dose parenteral MTX could improve clinical joint symptoms in PsA, albeit with a substantial risk of AEs.

Several subsequent observational open-label studies have supported the findings of Black and colleagues, demonstrating that MTX can lead to a clinical improvement in joint symptoms in PsA. In a single-center longitudinal observational study of 59 patients with PsA,[7] 68% exhibited a 40% or greater reduction in joint count. In that study, patients were treated with a mean MTX dose of 16.2 mg/wk for at least 24 months. Similarly, in an open-label randomized controlled trial of 35 patients with early PsA,[8] patients treated with MTX and nonsteroidal anti-inflammatory drug (NSAID) combination therapy had a greater improvement in their swollen and tender joint count compared with the NSAID monotherapy group at 3 months. These findings are echoed by Lie and colleagues[9], who published data on 430 patients with PsA treated with MTX monotherapy, collected as part of the Norwegian-DMARD registry. The mean MTX starting dose was 10.5 mg, increasing to 13.7 mg at 6 months. At 6 months, patients with PsA improved in most disease activity measures and patient reported outcomes. Comparing this with patients with RA treated with MTX in the same registry (n = 1218), patients with PsA tended to have less improvement, although changes were in the same range. Moreover, 65% of patients with PsA were maintained on MTX by 2 years, compared with 66% of patients with RA. However, the outcome measures used in this study were more relevant to RA than PsA, for example, the Disease Activity Score (DAS28).

Furthermore, there is also some evidence that MTX can lead to improvements in composite scores. Baranauskaite and colleagues[10] undertook the Remicade Study in Psoriatic Arthritis Patients Of Methotrexate-Naïve Disease (RESPOND) study, an open-label randomized controlled trial of 115 MTX-naive patients, comparing MTX monotherapy with MTX plus infliximab combination therapy. MTX was administered at a dose of 15 mg/wk. Although combination therapy with infliximab was found to be superior at 16 weeks, the ACR responses for the monotherapy group were relatively high: ACR20 66.7%, ACR50 39.6%, and ACR70 18.8%. Furthermore, 24.1% of patients also achieved MDA with MTX monotherapy. These findings are echoed in a post hoc analysis of MTX efficacy in the TICOPA study by Coates and Helliwell 2016.[11] The TICOPA study was an open-label multicenter randomized controlled trial comparing tight control of PsA versus standard care. Patients in the study had less than 24 months of symptom duration, and were DMARD naive. In the tight control arm, MTX monotherapy was the first DMARD used for the first 12 weeks unless contraindicated. MTX doses started at 15 mg/wk for 4 weeks then escalated to 25 mg/wk. In the standard care arm, MTX was used at the discretion of the treating physician. In the first 12 weeks of the trial, 188 patients received MTX, with 104 receiving a mean dose of greater than 15 mg/wk. The ACR outcomes at 12 weeks were: ACR20 40.8%, ACR50 18.8%, and ACR70 8.6%. Notably, there was a significant reduction in individual tender and swollen joints. Using the psoriatic arthritis disease activity score (PASDAS) response criteria, 57.4% achieved a moderate/good response, and 18.5% achieved a good response. Moreover, 22.4% of patients achieved MDA. Interestingly, there was a trend toward higher proportions of patients taking greater than 15 mg/wk of MTX achieving ACR20, ACR50, and a PASDAS moderate response. However, this is difficult to assess, because patients with well-controlled disease may be maintained on lower doses. Both RESPOND and TICOPA showed that MTX can improve joint outcomes in PsA, with approximately one-fifth of patients achieving MDA. However, both studies are limited by their open-label nature and lack of a placebo comparator. Indeed, a small double-blind placebo-controlled randomized controlled trial by Willkens and colleagues[12] found that MTX was superior to placebo in improving skin psoriasis and physician assessment of disease activity; however, it was not significantly better at improving joint swelling or tenderness, morning stiffness, or patient assessment of disease activity. This study recruited 37 patients with active peripheral PsA $\geq$6 months duration. MTX was given orally, at a dose of 7.5 to 15 mg/wk, spread over 3 doses.

In a recent phase 3 randomized multicenter double-blind study (Study of Etanercept and Methotrexate in Combination or as Monotherapy in Subjects with Psoriatic Arthritis [SEAM-PsA]) by Mease and colleagues,[13] 851 patients with active PsA, who were naive to MTX and biologics, were randomized into 3 groups: MTX monotherapy plus injectable placebo (n = 284), etanercept monotherapy plus oral placebo (n = 284), and MTX plus etanercept combination therapy (n = 283). In this cohort, the median PsA duration was 0.6 years (mean of 3.2 years). MTX was administered orally, at a dose of 20 mg/wk, and from week 4 to 24, the MTX-containing arms maintained a mean MTX dose greater than 18.8 mg. At 24 weeks, ACR responses for the MTX monotherapy group were: ACR20 50.7%, ACR50 30.6%, and ACR70 13.8%. A total of 22.9% of the MTX monotherapy group achieved MDA, with a mean decrease in PASDAS of 1.98 from baseline. Attainment of MDA has clinical significance, as it correlates with patients reporting low impact of disease, in addition to better functional and radiographic outcomes.[14–17]

In addition to evidence that MTX can lead to improved ACR outcomes and achievement of MDA, a study by Cantini and colleagues[18] also suggests that MTX can lead to remission in PsA. The authors analyzed 121 patients with PsA on MTX monotherapy, at a dose of 10 to 15 mg/wk. They used a very stringent definition of remission, which required the following criteria to be met: fatigue (visual analog scale [VAS] 1–100 mm) <10, pain (VAS 1–100 mm) <10, articular morning stiffness ≤15 minutes, tender joint count = 0, swollen joint count = 0, ESR ≤30 for women and 20 for men, C-reactive protein (CRP) ≤0.5, absent dactylitis, enthesitis/tenosynovitis, inflammatory spinal pain, and extra-articular features. There were 23 episodes of remission in patients on MTX monotherapy, demonstrating that remission with MTX is possible in a small number of patients. The ACR responses were AR20 41%, ACR50 28%, and ACR70 12%, respectively.

Despite the clinical improvement in symptoms seen with MTX, evidence from randomized controlled trials and observational studies suggest that MTX has limited disease-modifying effect in PsA. Scarpa and colleagues[8] conducted an open-label randomized controlled trial of 35 patients with early PsA, comparing NSAID monotherapy with NSAID plus MTX combination therapy. Although the MTX group had greater improvement in joint symptoms at 3 months, there was no difference between the 2 groups in terms of inflammatory markers, or patient and physician assessments of disease activity. Chandran and colleagues[7] published a single-center retrospective observational study of 59 patients with PsA treated with MTX for ≥24 months over a 10-year period. They found that, although two-thirds of patients demonstrated an improvement in skin and joint symptoms, there was nevertheless radiographic progression with a mean increase of 1.5 in the radiographic score using the modified Steinbrocker method. Interestingly, compared with a previous study in the same clinic,[19] Chandran and colleagues demonstrated that a greater proportion of patients achieved ≥40% reduction in joint counts (68% vs 47%), with reduced radiographic progression (1.5 vs 2.3) at 24 months. This was associated with MTX use earlier (mean disease duration 8 vs 11.5 years), and at higher doses of MTX (16.2 vs 10.8 mg/wk), which may account for better outcomes. However, a cohort analysis undertaken by Eder and colleagues[20] demonstrated again that MTX therapy does not halt radiographic progression in PsA, even if it does partially affect natural progression. Of 50 patients, 34 (68%) developed a new erosion in at least 1 joint and 40 (80%) had radiographic progression at 1 to 2 years using the modified Steinbrocker score. By 3 to 4 years, 42 (84%) patients had developed a new erosion in at least 1 joint, and 44 (88%) had radiographic progression. Similarly, SEAM-PsA[13] used the van der Heijde-modified Total Sharp Score, a different radiographic scoring system, to show that 10.6% of patients treated with MTX monotherapy had radiographic progression from baseline by week 48, with a mean change of 0.08.

Given the controversy surrounding the efficacy of MTX in PsA, the Methotrexate in Psoriatic Arthritis (MIPA)[21] trial was conducted, starting in 2003. Published in 2012, it is the largest randomized placebo-controlled trial of MTX in PsA to date. The authors compared MTX at a dose of 15 mg/wk to placebo in 221 patients with active peripheral PsA. The dose of MTX was increased slowly, from 7.5 mg/wk to 10 mg/wk at 4 weeks, and 15 mg/wk at 8 weeks. There was an option to increase the MTX dose to 20 mg/wk at 4 months, and 25 mg/wk at 5 months, at the discretion of the supervising rheumatologist. The primary outcome was the PsA response criteria (PsARC) at 6 months, which showed no significant effect with MTX compared with placebo (odds ratio [OR] = 1.77; 95% CI, 0.97, 3.23). Moreover, there was no significant effect of MTX compared with placebo on ACR20 (OR = 2.00; 95% CI, 0.65, 6.22) or DAS-28 (OR = 1.70; 95% CI, 0.90, 3.17). No significant treatment effect was observed for tender and swollen joints, ESR, CRP, Health Assessment Questionnaire, and pain. However, the MTX group did have a significant reduction in patient and assessor global scores and skin scores. The results of this study suggest that, although MTX improved skin disease and symptoms, it did not improve inflammatory synovitis and thus did not have a true disease-modifying effect. This study was one of the first to enroll a significant proportion of patients with oligoarthritis with only 1 active joint required at entry. Some of the lack of response may relate to poorer sensitivity of established outcome measures in this group. Supplementary data from the study support this, with much higher responses seen in polyarticular patients (n = 142) compared with patients with oligoarthritis (n = 79). There are a few limitations to this trial, including a long recruitment time, mild disease at entry, low-dose MTX with slow up-titration, high drop-out rate, and limited statistical power. There is also a lack of radiographic data to assess radiographic progression between MTX- and placebo-treated patients. Furthermore, although the trial examined peripheral arthritis and skin and nail disease, it failed to assess other domains within PsA such as enthesitis, dactylitis, and axial involvement.

Kane and colleagues[22] investigated the effect of MTX on synovial inflammation and gene expression in PsA, through synovial biopsies of an inflamed knee pre-MTX and post-MTX treatment in 10 patients with active PsA. MTX was administered orally, with a median dose of 13.75 mg/wk. The median interval between synovial biopsies was 11.5 months. Post-MTX, there was a significant reduction in the Ritchie Articular Index, swollen joint count, and Disease Activity Score, which corresponded to a significant decrease in CD3, CD4, CD8, CD68, E-selectin, and intercellular adhesion molecule immunohistochemical staining. Moreover, decreased proinflammatory cytokine expression was observed, however the effect was only significant for interleukin-8. Despite a significant reduction in synovial thickness, synovial hypervascularity was not significantly reduced and there remained a residual T cell infiltrate in all synovial biopsy tissues post-MTX. Taken together, these results suggest that MTX reduces, but does not abolish, synovial inflammation in PsA.

As MTX seems to have a beneficial effect in PsA in those who respond, Chandran and colleagues[23] investigated the genetic predictors of MTX efficacy in a longitudinal cohort of patients with PsA. Using response to MTX at 6 months as a cutoff, they classified patients who achieved a ≥50% decrease in active inflamed joint count from baseline as responders. A total of 119 patients were included in the effectiveness analysis, with a mean age of 44.1, mean duration of PsA of 9.3 years, and mean number of 15.5 actively inflamed joints. In this cohort, the authors tested 5 single nucleotide polymorphisms in genes involved in the folate pathway (MTHFR 677T, MTHFR 1298C, DHFR −473T, DHFR 35289A, and RFC 80A) for association for MTX response. Using logistic regression and adjusting for concomitant medications, only the minor A allele of DHFR gene at +35289 was associated with increased odds of MTX response after 6 months of therapy (OR = 2.99; 95% CI, 1.20, 7.55). MTX inhibits DHFR, which converts dihydrofolate to tetrahydrofolate. This study suggests there may be a genetic element to MTX response in PsA.

Should we use methotrexate to treat peripheral arthritis in PsA? There is a paucity of high-quality data from randomized controlled trials on the efficacy of MTX in treating peripheral arthritis in PsA. Available data are often derived from old studies, studies with small sample sizes or poor design, and studies limited by their observational nature with lack of appropriate controls. A recent Cochrane systematic review of 8 trials concluded that there is only low-quality evidence for the efficacy of low-dose ($\leq$15 mg) oral MTX compared with placebo when taken for 6 months, in terms of PsARC, function, pain, and patient and physician global assessments of disease activity.[24] Studies thus far suggest that MTX use earlier in the disease process with higher doses seems to be associated with improved outcomes, and in a small proportion of patients, it is possible to achieve MDA. However, MTX therapy does not abolish radiographic progression or synovial inflammation, suggesting that it may not fully halt the underlying disease process.

When considering the efficacy of other csDMARDs in PsA, there is also a relative lack of data. Clegg and colleagues[25] compared sulfasalazine (SSZ) with placebo in a pivotal randomized controlled trial of 221 patients with PsA. Although they showed that patients on SSZ had significantly higher response rates compared with placebo, the overall response rate for SSZ was not particularly high, at 57.8%. In a subsequent Cochrane review meta-analysis,[26] the authors concluded that SSZ was effective in PsA but with a small effect size. Kaltwasser and colleagues[27] published the results of the Treatment of Psoriatic Arthritis Study group, which compared leflunomide (LFN) to placebo in 190 patients with active PsA and psoriasis. At 24 weeks, the LFN group had significantly higher response rates as measured by the PsARC compared with placebo, with similar trends observed for ARC20 and PASI (Psoriasis Area and Severity Index) responses. However, LFN is not frequently used in clinical practice, with concerns over rare but serious adverse effects on the liver. Moreover, patients frequently do not tolerate the drug well.

There are limited data on the relative efficacy of different csDMARDs. In a single-center retrospective analysis of 53 patients with PsA on MTX, SSZ, and LFN,[28] all 3 agents led to consistent improvement in disease activity scores. However, SSZ seemed to exhibit greater efficacy compared with the other agents. The difficulties surrounding selecting the optimal csDMARD is reflected in the recent European League Against Rheumatism (EULAR) and Group for Research and Assessment of Psoriasis and Psoriatic Arthritis (GRAPPA) guidelines for the treatment of PsA.[29,30] Although both sets of guidelines advocate that in most cases, a csDMARD should be the initial step in therapy, the recommendations are different. EULAR recommends MTX as the preferred option, with SSZ or LFN considered if there are contraindications to MTX. In contrast, GRAPPA advocates starting MTX, SSZ, or LFN with no particular preference.

Moreover, there is clear evidence that biologics are superior to MTX in the treatment of PsA. In the RESPOND study,[10] a significantly higher proportion of patients receiving combination therapy with infliximab plus MTX achieved ACR20 by week 16 compared with patients on MTX monotherapy. In the SEAM-PsA study,[13] ACR20 and MDA response rates were significantly higher for patients on the etanercept monotherapy group compared with those on the MTX monotherapy group. These findings are echoed in a systematic literature review of randomized controlled trials by Kingsley and Scott,[31] which conclude that biologic agents seem to be more beneficial compared with csDMARDs. Indeed, the recently published American College of Rheumatology guidelines[32] for treatment of PsA advocates starting a tumor necrosis factor inhibitor (TNFi) biologic as first-line, rather than csDMARDs, due to their increased efficacy. This reflects a paradigm shift in the approach to treating peripheral PsA, as previously treatment with TNFi was viewed as a "step-up" option once treatment with csDMARDs fail.

Dactylitis and Enthesitis

There are very limited data on the efficacy of MTX to treat dactylitis and enthesitis in PsA as these domains have not been assessed well in older studies, and there are no data from placebo-controlled studies. In an open-label observational study of 28 patients with active PsA and new-onset dactylitis, Healy and Helliwell[33] assessed the impact of changing disease-modifying therapy on dactylitis. Although most patients were initiated on MTX (19/28), the results are not presented per treatment but for the cohort, which also includes patients on LFN, etanercept, and hydroxychloroquine. At 3 and 6 months, the cohort exhibited an improvement in dactylitis across multiple measures used for dactylitis, including the Leeds Dactylitis Index (LDI) basic. This corresponded to a PsARC and ACR20 response of 54% and 50% at 3 months, and of 51% and 43% at 6 months, respectively. Given that the data for patients on MTX are not separately presented and the lack of controls, it is difficult to draw robust conclusions. However, the results do tentatively suggest that MTX may improve dactylitis in patients with PsA.

As part of the post hoc analysis on the efficacy of MTX in PsA within the TICOPA study, Coates and Helliwell[11] also examined the effect of MTX on dactylitis and enthesitis. At 12 weeks, there was a significant reduction in the LDI basic score of 62.7% ($P = .033$), with complete resolution of dactylitis seen in 37/59 patients. Only 9 new cases of dactylitis were identified in patients without baseline involvement. In contrast, the median change in the enthesitis score was 0, independent of whether the Leeds Enthesitis Index, the Infliximab Multinational Psoriatic Arthritis Controlled Trial (IMPACT) enthesitis score, or the Maastricht Ankylosing Spondylitis Enthesitis Score was used. However, 38/148 patients had resolution of symptoms, with only 8 new cases of enthesitis identified, which were not present at baseline. At 12 weeks, the proportions of patients with dactylitis and enthesitis were both significantly lower compared with baseline.

Similarly, in SEAM-PsA,[13] the authors observed an improvement in dactylitis and enthesitis in the MTX monotherapy arm within the SEAM-PsA study. Using the LDI, 34.5% of patients had an LDI greater than 0 at baseline. At 24 weeks, the mean change (SE) from baseline was −128.8 (26.8), with 65.2% of patients having resolution of dactylitis. Using the Spondyloarthritis Research Consortium of Canada (SPARCC) enthesitis index, 67.3% of patients had a score >0 at baseline. At 24 weeks, the mean change from baseline was −3.1, with 43.1% of patients with enthesitis experiencing resolution. Collectively, these results indicate that MTX may exert a beneficial effect on dactylitis and enthesitis in patients with PsA.

Should we use methotrexate to treat dactylitis and enthesitis in PsA? Overall, there is very limited evidence for the efficacy of MTX and other csDMARDs in the treatment of dactylitis and enthesitis. In the SSZ study by Clegg and colleagues,[25] there was no significant difference in the dactylitis and enthesitis scores between patients treated with SSZ and placebo. In patients with predominantly entheseal disease, current guidelines[29,30,32] recommend starting with biologic agents as the initial step rather than using MTX and other csDMARDs, as more robust evidence is available for biologics. However, this approach may need to be reconsidered given the recent results of the SEAM-PsA study,[13] which demonstrated no significant difference in the LDI and SPARCC enthesitis index between the etanercept monotherapy and MTX monotherapy groups at 24 weeks.

Axial Disease

MTX and other traditional csDMARDS are not effective in axial PsA, and thus MTX is not used to treat axial disease. Although no existing studies have examined the use of MTX in axial PsA, a recent Cochrane Systematic Review[34] has been published summarising the evidence in ankylosing spondylitis (AS). The authors identified 3 randomized controlled trials in 116 participants with AS, and concluded that there was insufficient evidence to suggest that MTX therapy provided benefit in the treatment of AS.

Moreover, current measures of axial disease such as the Bath Ankylosing Spondylitis Disease Activity Index (BASDAI) does not discriminate well between peripheral and axial PsA. Taylor and Harrison[35] studied 2 samples of patients with PsA, one from a disease register (n = 133), and one from consecutive clinic attendees (n = 47), and found that the BASDAI does not discriminate well between axial and peripheral PsA. Fernáandez-Sueiro and colleagues[36] compared the BASDAI scores between 54 patients with peripheral PsA, 46 with axial PsA and 103 with primary AS. They found similar BASDAI scores in axial and peripheral PsA, corroborating the findings of Taylor and Harrison.[35] The lack of a measure that discriminates between axial and peripheral disease within PsA poses challenges in clinical trials focusing on axial disease, as it is difficult to differentiate whether changes in outcomes are due to axial disease or other disease domains within PsA.

Psoriasis

MTX has consistently been shown to be effective in treating psoriasis, and is recommended as the first-line systemic csDMARD for moderate to severe psoriasis in European and US guidelines.[37,38] A recent meta-analysis of 11 studies by West and colleagues[39] found that approximately 45% of patients with psoriasis on MTX achieve PASI 75 by 12 or 16 weeks compared with 4.4% of patients in the placebo group. However, there was substantial heterogeneity between the studies, with an I^2 of 92.7%. The authors conclude that although it seems that MTX is effective in treating psoriasis, it is difficult to quantify exactly how effective it is.

As most studies of MTX efficacy in psoriasis utilize oral preparations, Warren and colleagues[40] published the MTX in patients with moderate to severe plaque-type psoriasis (METOP) study, which focuses on the efficacy of subcutaneous MTX in psoriasis. The rationale behind subcutaneous administration is based on previous observations that patients with poor response to oral MTX may benefit from subcutaneous MTX.[41] These findings corroborate a study in RA[42] that showed superiority of subcutaneous MTX over oral MTX after 24 weeks. The METOP study is a multicenter randomized double-blind placebo-controlled phase 3 trial investigating subcutaneous MTX in patients with moderate to severe plaque-type psoriasis. One hundred and twenty MTX-naive patients with a diagnosis of chronic plaque psoriasis for $\geq$6 months, and moderate to severe disease at baseline were randomized into receiving either subcutaneous MTX at a dose of 17.5 mg/wk (n = 91) or placebo (n = 29) for the first 16 weeks. At 8 weeks, the dose of subcutaneous MTX could be increased to 22.5 mg/wk if there had not been $\geq$50% reduction in baseline PASI. After 16 weeks, the study became open-label, with all patients receiving MTX up to 52 weeks. At 16 weeks, a significantly higher proportion of patients in the MTX group achieved a PASI 75 response compared with placebo (41% vs 10%, risk ratio = 3.93; 95% CI, 1.31–11.91; *P* = .0026). At 52 weeks, there was no significant difference between the proportions of patients achieving a PASI 75 response between the 2 groups, with all patients receiving MTX. Paired baseline and week 16 skin biopsies were available for 27 patients (placebo = 6, MTX PASI 75 nonresponders = 7, MTX PASI 75 responders = 14). Interestingly, MTX responders had prominent reductions in the numbers of skin-infiltrating CD3-positive T cells and CD11c-positive dendritic cells, with week 16 numbers almost returning to values in normal skin. Moreover, MTX responders had reduced cutaneous mRNA levels of IL17A at week 16, whereas in MTX nonresponders and placebo this was not significantly changed. Collectively, these results illustrate that subcutaneous MTX is efficacious in treating psoriasis, and also sheds light on the potential immunomodulatory mechanisms underlying the clinical response to MTX in psoriasis. However, the question of whether subcutaneous MTX is more efficacious compared with oral MTX in psoriasis remains unanswered.

In patients with PsA, MTX remains effective in treating psoriasis. In the MIPA trial,[21] linear regression analysis showed that the MTX group had a significant reduction in PASI compared with placebo. In the post hoc analysis of the TICOPA trial,[11] 158 patients had psoriasis and 27.2% of patients were able to achieve a PASI 75 response by week 12. In the MTX monotherapy group in SEAM-PsA,[13] 66.1% of patients with ≥3% body surface area affected at baseline had an improvement by 24 weeks. Similarly, 65.7% of patients with ≥10% body surface area affected at baseline had an improvement by 24 weeks.

Nail Disease

Compared with psoriasis, there is very limited evidence for MTX in the treatment of psoriatic nail disease. Moreover, the available evidence is limited by the short follow-up duration. The MIPA study[21] did not find a treatment effect in either the MTX group or the placebo group at 3 and 6 months. In the TICOPA study,[11] 117 patients had nail involvement. At 12 weeks, the median change in modified Nail Psoriasis Severity Index (mNAPSI) score was −2 (interquartile range −8, 0), the median change in the nail plate score was 0 (interquartile range −3.75, 1), and the median change in the nail bed score was −1 (interquartile range −4.75, 0). In the study by Mease and colleagues,[13] 65.1% of patients in the MTX monotherapy group had a mNAPSI greater than 0 at baseline. At 24 weeks, the mean change from baseline was −1.1, with 38.8% of patients achieving a score of 1. The METOP study[40] also examined the effect of MTX on nail psoriasis, using the NAPSI score of the worst fingernail as the target nail. At 16 weeks, the MTX group had a reduced NAPSI score, compared with no change in the placebo group. At 52 weeks, complete clearance of nail disease was seen in 14% of patients with active nail psoriasis at baseline. These results suggest that MTX may have a beneficial effect in nail disease. However, the response is likely to be slow, due to the slowing of nail growth.

METHOTREXATE AND BIOLOGICS COMBINATION THERAPY

MTX is frequently used in combination with TNFi; however, it is unclear whether this leads to better outcomes. Saad and colleagues[43] conducted an observational study of 595 patients with PsA from the British Society for Rheumatology Biologics Register. At 6 months, they found similar EULAR response rates in patients receiving TNFi monotherapy (79.5%), TNFi in combination with MTX (78.1%), and TNFi in combination with another DMARD (73.3%). Fagerli and colleagues[44] compared TNFi and MTX combination therapy (n = 270) to TNFi monotherapy (n = 170) in an observational study using the NOR-DMARD registry. In the combination therapy group, the mean MTX dose was 14.7 mg. At 3 and 6 months, the authors observed minimal differences between the 2 groups in the change in the physician and patient global scores.

Looking only at patients with ≥1 swollen joint at baseline, there was also no difference between the 2 groups in the change in DAS28 and disease activity in psoriatic arthritis at 3 and 6 months. Interestingly, the combination therapy group had a trend toward improved drug survival at 3 years compared with the monotherapy group, with the results being most marked for infliximab. Moreover, the TNFi monotherapy group had an increased frequency of AEs, and also had a higher percentage discontinuing for loss or lack of efficacy compared with the combination therapy group. This therefore suggests that although concomitant MTX use with TNFi does not improve outcomes it may, however, improve TNFi survival.

MTX monotherapy, etanercept monotherapy, and MTX plus etanercept combination therapy were compared in the SEAM-PsA trial,[13] a phase 3 double-blind randomized controlled trial of 851 patients with PsA naive to both MTX and biologics. At week 24, ACR20 and MDA responses were similar between the etanercept monotherapy and combination therapy groups (ACR20: 60.9% vs 65.0%, MDA: 35.9% vs 35.7%). These findings corroborate results in previous studies, suggesting that concomitant MTX use does not improve outcomes compared with TNFi monotherapy. However, further studies with other TNFi biologics are required to investigate whether MTX improves TNFi survival, given that etanercept, as a fusion protein, may behave differently to other monoclonal antibodies in terms of long-term drug survival and risk of immunogenicity.

MTX is also frequently used in combination with other non-TNFi biologics in the treatment of PsA, for example, secukinumab, ustekinumab, and tofacitinib. A pooled analysis of 2049 patients from 4 phase 3 studies on secukinumab in patients with PsA showed no clear difference between efficacy outcomes in patients with and without concomitant MTX use.[45] A retrospective analysis of 487 episodes of ustekinumab treatment in patients with PsA in Hungary showed that concomitant MTX did not have a significant effect on ustekinumab survival.[46] These results suggest that perhaps concomitant MTX use does not improve non-TNFi biologic efficacy or survival; however, further research is required to support this given there is only very limited evidence available at present.

SURVIVAL, TOLERABILITY, AND ADVERSE EVENTS

At present very few studies have examined the survival of MTX in patients with PsA. A single-center retrospective Brazilian study of 161 patients with PsA treated with TNFi and/or csDMARDs concluded that MTX has a shorter survival compared with TNFi.[47] At 6 and 12 months, 50.0% and 34.4% patients remained on MTX, compared with 83.4% and 66.4% on TNFi, respectively. In a single-center retrospective study in the UK, involving 762 patients with RA and 193 patients with PsA, the median duration of MTX treatment was 10 months for both groups.[48] They identified that the 2 most common reasons for discontinuation were adverse effects (RA, 77.5%; PsA, 62.0%) and inefficacy (RA, 12.4%; PsA, 18.3%). In patients with PsA who discontinued MTX due to adverse effects, the most common reasons were gastrointestinal symptoms (27.3%), abnormal liver function tests (27.3%), and respiratory symptoms (13.6%). Only 1 patient discontinued due to neutropenia. At time of MTX discontinuation, the mean MTX in patients with PsA was 13.6 mg/wk.

In the MIPA trial,[21] common AEs, defined as greater than 5% within a treatment arm, were nausea and vomiting, respiratory tract infections, and abnormal liver function tests. In the TICOPA study,[11] the most common AEs reported were nausea, fatigue, and liver abnormalities. Of 188 patients, only 14 discontinued MTX due to an adverse event (fatigue, 1; nausea, 5; gastrointestinal symptoms, 1; headache/migraine, 1; liver

Box 1
Summary of evidence for the use of methotrexate (MTX) in PsA

Area	Summary of Evidence
Peripheral arthritis	• Evidence from randomized controlled trials and open-label studies suggest that MTX may improve joint symptoms in peripheral arthritis, with associated improvements in global scores.[6–9,21] However, the overall quality of the evidence is low, as concluded by a recent Cochrane systematic review.[24] • Three recent randomized controlled trials have shown that approximately one-fifth of patients with PsA on MTX achieve MDA.[10,11,13] However, this needs to be interpreted with caution due to lack of a placebo comparator. • MTX use earlier in the disease process, at higher doses, seems to be associated with improved outcomes.[7] • There are limited data on the relative efficacy of MTX compared with other csDMARDs, as reflected by variation in current guidelines on the preferred initial csDMARD.[29,30]
Radiographic progression	• Observational studies have shown that MTX does not halt radiographic progression.[7,13,20] However, higher doses used earlier in the disease process are associated with less radiographic progression.[7] • A recent randomized controlled trial has shown that etanercept use is associated with significantly lower rates of radiographic progression compared with MTX.[13] • The overall quality of the evidence is very low.
Enthesitis	• Two studies have shown that MTX use may be associated with improvements in enthesitis in patients with PsA; however, both studies lack a placebo comparator.[11,13] • Current guidelines recommend using biologic agents as the first-line treatment in patients with predominantly entheseal disease, rather than MTX and other csDMARDs.[29,30,32] • The overall quality of the evidence is very low.
Dactylitis	• Two studies have shown that MTX use may be associated with improvements in dactylitis in patients with PsA; however, both studies lack a placebo comparator.[11,13] • The overall quality of the evidence is very low.
Axial disease	• MTX does not seem to be effective in axial PsA.
Psoriasis	• Evidence from randomized controlled trials and observational studies suggest that MTX is effective at treating psoriasis, with 27%–45% of patients achieving PASI75 at 12–16 wk.[13,21,39,40]
Nail disease	• MTX may have a beneficial effect in nail disease, with 1 study showing a reduction in the NAPSI score of the MTX group compared with placebo.[40] • The overall quality of the evidence is very low, due to limited numbers of studies with short follow-up durations.
Coprescription with biologics	• Randomized controlled trials and observational studies have shown that coprescription of MTX and biologics does not seem to lead to improved outcomes. However, concurrent MTX use may improve TNFi survival.[13,43,44] • The overall quality of the evidence is low.
Adverse effects	• Adverse effects are a common reason for MTX discontinuation, with gastrointestinal symptoms and abnormal liver function tests as the most common reasons.[45]

Abbreviations: csDMARD, conventional synthetic disease-modifying antirheumatic drug; MDA, minimal disease activity; PASI, psoriasis area and severity index; TNFi, tumor necrosis factor inhibitor.

abnormalities, 4), although the MTX dose was modified or temporarily suspended in 77 patients. In a recent Cochrane systematic review of the use of MTX in PsA, the authors concluded that it remains uncertain whether MTX causes more harm than placebo, due to the small numbers of reported AEs.[24]

SUMMARY

MTX is widely used in the treatment of PsA; however, there is limited evidence for its efficacy in multiple domains (**Box 1**). There is a paucity of comparative studies and strategy trials, which explains the differences between treatment recommendations for the initial step in PsA treatment. Some advocate MTX and other csDMARDs as the initial choice, whereas others advocate starting TNFi. There is no clear evidence for whether delaying access to biologics affects outcomes, and there is limited evidence on the optimal treatments in early disease. Given the heterogeneous nature of psoriatic disease, a personalized approach is required when deciding on the most appropriate therapy for individual patients.

It is clear that MTX is effective in skin psoriasis. It seems likely that MTX may improve joint symptoms in peripheral arthritis, with earlier use and higher initial doses being linked to better outcomes. MTX may also have a beneficial effect in dactylitis, enthesitis, and psoriatic nail disease, but it is likely to exert a limited immunomodulatory effect rather than fully halting the disease process. Most studies on MTX in PsA are old and small scale with poor study designs, which limits the quality of the evidence. More recent studies have provided increasing evidence for the effectiveness of MTX in PsA; however, these are not placebo controlled.

Using MTX in combination with a TNFi does not seem to improve outcomes; however it may increase TNFi survival. Moreover, MTX is generally well tolerated, with the main adverse effects being gastrointestinal symptoms and liver abnormalities. However, over time, a relatively small number of people remain on MTX monotherapy either due to lack of efficacy or intolerable side effects. Although MTX is less effective than the newer biologic therapies in treating PsA,[13] it is cheap and widely accessible, and therefore likely to retain an important role in the management of PsA, especially in more resource-limited health care settings.

REFERENCES

1. Van den Bosch F, Coates L. Clinical management of psoriatic arthritis. Lancet 2018;391(10136):2285–94.
2. Coates LC, Moverley AR, McParland L, et al. Effect of tight control of inflammation in early psoriatic arthritis (TICOPA): a UK multicentre, open-label, randomised controlled trial. Lancet 2015;386(10012):2489–98.
3. Coates LC, Fransen J, Helliwell PS. Defining minimal disease activity in psoriatic arthritis: a proposed objective target for treatment. Ann Rheum Dis 2010;69(01): 48–53.
4. Ceponis A, Kavanaugh A. Use of methotrexate in patients with psoriatic arthritis. Clin Exp Rheumatol 2010;28(5 Suppl 61):S132–7.
5. Elmamoun M, Chandran V. Role of methotrexate in the management of psoriatic arthritis. Drugs 2018;78(6):611–9.
6. Black RL, O'Brien WM, Scott EJV, et al. Methotrexate therapy in psoriatic arthritis: double-blind study on 21 patients. JAMA 1964;189(10):743–7.
7. Chandran V, Schentag CT, Gladman DD. Reappraisal of the effectiveness of methotrexate in psoriatic arthritis: results from a longitudinal observational cohort. J Rheumatol 2008;35(3):469–71.
8. Scarpa R, Peluso R, Atteno M, et al. The effectiveness of a traditional therapeutical approach in early psoriatic arthritis: results of a pilot randomised 6-month trial with methotrexate. Clin Rheumatol 2008;27(7):823–6.

9. Lie E, van der Heijde D, Uhlig T, et al. Effectiveness and retention rates of methotrexate in psoriatic arthritis in comparison with methotrexate-treated patients with rheumatoid arthritis. Ann Rheum Dis 2010;69(4):671–6.
10. Baranauskaite A, Raffayová H, Kungurov NV, et al. Infliximab plus methotrexate is superior to methotrexate alone in the treatment of psoriatic arthritis in methotrexate-naive patients: the RESPOND study. Ann Rheum Dis 2012;71(4): 541–8.
11. Coates LC, Helliwell PS. Methotrexate efficacy in the tight control in psoriatic arthritis study. J Rheumatol 2016;43(2):356–61.
12. Willkens RF, Williams HJ, Ward JR, et al. Randomized, double-blind, placebo controlled trial of low-dose pulse methotrexate in psoriatic arthritis. Arthritis Rheum 1984;27(4):376–81.
13. Mease PJ, Gladman DD, Collier DH, et al. Etanercept and methotrexate as monotherapy or in combination for psoriatic arthritis: primary results from a randomized, controlled phase 3 trial. Arthritis Rheumatol 2019. https://doi.org/10.1002/art.40851.
14. Coates LC, Helliwell PS. Validation of minimal disease activity criteria for psoriatic arthritis using interventional trial data. Arthritis Care Res (Hoboken) 2010;62: 965–9.
15. Coates LC, Cook R, Lee KA, et al. Frequency, predictors, and prognosis of sustained minimal disease activity in an observational psoriatic arthritis cohort. Arthritis Care Res (Hoboken) 2010;62:970–6.
16. Kavanaugh A, van der Heijde D, Beutler A, et al. Radiographic progression of patients with psoriatic arthritis who achieve minimal disease activity in response to golimumab therapy: results through 5 years of a randomized, placebo-controlled study. Arthritis Care Res (Hoboken) 2016;68:267–74.
17. Queiro R, Canete JD, Montilla C, et al. Minimal disease activity and impact of disease in psoriatic arthritis: a Spanish cross-sectional multicenter study. Arthritis Res Ther 2017;19:72.
18. Cantini F, Niccoli L, Nannini C, et al. Frequency and duration of clinical remission in patients with peripheral psoriatic arthritis requiring second-line drugs. Rheumatology (Oxford) 2008;47(6):872–6.
19. Abu-Shakra M, Gladman DD, Thorne JC, et al. Longterm methotrexate therapy in psoriatic arthritis: clinical and radiological outcome. J Rheumatol 1995;22(2): 241–5.
20. Eder L, Thavaneswaran A, Chandran V, et al. Tumour necrosis factor α blockers are more effective than methotrexate in the inhibition of radiographic joint damage progression among patients with psoriatic arthritis. Ann Rheum Dis 2014; 73(6):1007–11.
21. Kingsley GH, Kowalczyk A, Taylor H, et al. A randomized placebo-controlled trial of methotrexate in psoriatic arthritis. Rheumatology (Oxford) 2012;51(8):1368–77.
22. Kane D, Gogarty M, O'leary J, et al. Reduction of synovial sublining layer inflammation and proinflammatory cytokine expression in psoriatic arthritis treated with methotrexate. Arthritis Rheum 2004;50(10):3286–95.
23. Chandran V, Siannis F, Rahman P, et al. Folate pathway enzyme gene polymorphisms and the efficacy and toxicity of methotrexate in psoriatic arthritis. J Rheumatol 2010;37(7):1508–12.
24. Wilsdon TD, Whittle SL, Thynne TR, et al. Methotrexate for psoriatic arthritis. Cochrane Database Syst Rev 2019;(1):CD012722.

25. Clegg DO, Reda DJ, Weisman MH, et al. Comparison of sulfasalazine and placebo in the treatment of ankylosing spondylitis. A department of veterans affairs cooperative study. Arthritis Rheum 1996;39(12):2004–12.
26. Jones G, Crotty M, Brooks P. Interventions for psoriatic arthritis. Cochrane Database Syst Rev 2000;(3):CD000212.
27. Kaltwasser JP, Nash P, Gladman D, et al. Efficacy and safety of leflunomide in the treatment of psoriatic arthritis and psoriasis: a multinational, double-blind, randomized, placebo-controlled clinical trial. Arthritis Rheum 2004;50(6):1939–50.
28. Roussou E, Bouraoui A. Real-life experience of using conventional disease-modifying anti-rheumatic drugs (DMARDs) in psoriatic arthritis (PsA). Retrospective analysis of the efficacy of methotrexate, sulfasalazine, and leflunomide in PsA in comparison to spondyloarthritides other than PsA and literature review of the use of conventional DMARDs in PsA. Eur J Rheumatol 2017;4(1):1–10.
29. Gossec L, Smolen JS, Ramiro S, et al. European league against rheumatism (EULAR) recommendations for the management of psoriatic arthritis with pharmacological therapies: 2015 update. Ann Rheum Dis 2016;75(3):499–510.
30. Coates LC, Kavanaugh A, Mease PJ, et al. Group for research and assessment of psoriasis and psoriatic arthritis 2015 treatment recommendations for psoriatic arthritis. Arthritis Rheumatol 2016;68(5):1060–71.
31. Kingsley GH, Scott DL. Assessing the effectiveness of synthetic and biologic disease-modifying antirheumatic drugs in psoriatic arthritis - a systematic review. Psoriasis (Auckl) 2015;5:71–81.
32. Singh JA, Guyatt G, Ogdie A, et al. Special article: 2018 American College of Rheumatology/National Psoriasis Foundation guideline for the treatment of psoriatic arthritis. Arthritis Care Res (Hoboken) 2019;71(1):2–29.
33. Healy PJ, Helliwell PS. Measuring dactylitis in clinical trials: which is the best instrument to use? J Rheumatol 2007;34(6):1302–6.
34. Chen J, Veras MMS, Liu C, et al. Methotrexate for ankylosing spondylitis. Cochrane Database Syst Rev 2013;(2):CD004524.
35. Taylor WJ, Harrison AA. Could the bath ankylosing spondylitis disease activity index (BASDAI) be a valid measure of disease activity in patients with psoriatic arthritis? Arthritis Rheum 2004;51(3):311–5.
36. Fernández-Sueiro JL, Willisch A, Pértega-Díaz S, et al. Validity of the bath ankylosing spondylitis disease activity index for the evaluation of disease activity in axial psoriatic arthritis. Arthritis Care Res (Hoboken) 2010;62(1):78–85.
37. Psoriasis. Recommendations for methotrexate | American Academy of Dermatology. Available at: https://www.aad.org/practicecenter/quality/clinical-guidelines/psoriasis/systemic-agents/recommendations-for-methotrexate. Accessed January 13, 2019.
38. Warren RB, Weatherhead SC, Smith CH, et al. British Association of Dermatologists' guidelines for the safe and effective prescribing of methotrexate for skin disease 2016. Br J Dermatol 2016;175(1):23–44.
39. West J, Ogston S, Foerster J. Safety and efficacy of methotrexate in psoriasis: a meta-analysis of published trials. PLoS One 2016;11(5):e0153740.
40. Warren RB, Mrowietz U, von Kiedrowski R, et al. An intensified dosing schedule of subcutaneous methotrexate in patients with moderate to severe plaque-type psoriasis (METOP): a 52 week, multicentre, randomised, double-blind, placebo-controlled, phase 3 trial. Lancet 2017;389(10068):528–37.
41. Yesudian PD, Leman J, Balasubramaniam P, et al. Effectiveness of subcutaneous methotrexate in chronic plaque psoriasis. J Drugs Dermatol 2016;15(3):345–9.

42. Braun J, Kästner P, Flaxenberg P, et al. Comparison of the clinical efficacy and safety of subcutaneous versus oral administration of methotrexate in patients with active rheumatoid arthritis: results of a six-month, multicenter, randomized, double-blind, controlled, phase IV trial. Arthritis Rheum 2008;58:73–81.
43. Saad AA, Ashcroft DM, Watson KD, et al. Efficacy and safety of anti-TNF therapies in psoriatic arthritis: an observational study from the British Society for Rheumatology Biologics Register. Rheumatology (Oxford) 2010;49(4):697–705.
44. Fagerli KM, Lie E, van der Heijde D, et al. The role of methotrexate co-medication in TNF-inhibitor treatment in patients with psoriatic arthritis: results from 440 patients included in the NOR-DMARD study. Ann Rheum Dis 2014;73(1):132–7.
45. Kirkham B, Mease P, Nash P, et al. AB0945 Secukinumab efficacy in patients with active psoriatic arthritis: pooled analysis of four phase 3 trials by prior anti-tnf therapy and concomitant methotrexate use. Ann Rheum Dis 2018;77:1597–8.
46. Pogácsás L, Borsi A, Takács P, et al. Long-term drug survival and predictor analysis of the whole psoriatic patient population on biological therapy in Hungary. J Dermatolog Treat 2017;28(7):635–41.
47. Ribeiro da Silva MR, Ribeiro dos Santos JB, Maciel Almeida A, et al. Medication persistence for psoriatic arthritis in a Brazilian real-world setting. Future Sci OA 2019;5(2):FSO369.
48. Nikiphorou E, Negoescu A, Fitzpatrick JD, et al. Indispensable or intolerable? Methotrexate in patients with rheumatoid and psoriatic arthritis: a retrospective review of discontinuation rates from a large UK cohort. Clin Rheumatol 2014;33(5):609–14.

Is There a Role for MRI to Establish Treatment Indications and Effectively Monitor Response in Patients with Axial Spondyloarthritis?

Monica Schwartzman, MD[a,*],
Walter P. Maksymowych, MD, FRCP(C)[b]

KEYWORDS

• Spondyloarthritis • Sacroiliitis • Ankylosing spondylitis
• Magnetic resonance imaging • Radiography

KEY POINTS

- MRI detects lesions earlier than radiographs, which allows for the early identification of axial spondyloarthritis (axSpA) and prompt initiation of treatment.
- Spinal MRI findings in the absence of radiographic or MRI sacroiliac joint findings are uncommon and may impair specificity for the diagnosis of axSpA
- Adding spine MRI to the axSpA classification criteria captures only a few additional patients who would otherwise not be classified as axSpA
- MRI bone marrow edema is very sensitive for the evaluation of axSpA, although specificity remains a challenge as ASAS-defined active sacroiliitis can be seen in healthy individuals, postpartum women, and patients with mechanical disorders.
- There is literature supporting MRI as a prognostic tool in predicting radiographic progression of disease in the sacroiliac joint and spine.

Disclosure: W.P. Maksymowych has received honoraria and/or consulting fees from Abbvie, Boehringer, Celgene, Galapagos, Janssen, Lilly, Novartis, Pfizer, and UCB, and research and/or educational grants from Abbvie, Janssen, Novartis, Pfizer, and UCB. M. Schwartzman has no financial disclosures to report.
[a] Department of Medicine, Division of Rheumatology, The Hospital for Special Surgery, 535 East 70th Street 7th Floor, New York, NY 10021, USA; [b] Department of Medicine, Division of Rheumatology, University of Alberta, 568A Heritage Medical Research Centre, Edmonton, Alberta T6G2R3, Canada
* Corresponding author.
E-mail address: Schwartzmanm@hss.edu

Rheum Dis Clin N Am 45 (2019) 341–358
https://doi.org/10.1016/j.rdc.2019.04.009 rheumatic.theclinics.com

THE USE OF MRI IN AXIAL SPONDYLOARTHRITIS

Recognizing axial spondyloarthritis (axSpA) early in its disease course is challenging and diagnosis is often made long after symptoms start.[1] Radiography can detect disease; however, often years after the onset of symptoms. It is accepted that MRI can identify disease much earlier, even in the absence of radiographically evident disease.[2] As MRI has become more ubiquitous in clinical orthopedic and rheumatologic practice, its use in axSpA has become more frequent, particularly in the detection of early disease.

In 2009, the Assessment in Spondyloarthritis International Society (ASAS)-Outcome Measures in Rheumatology (OMERACT) MRI working group published a consensus-based definition for MRI-defined sacroiliitis for classification purposes.[3] In this definition, fulfilling the imaging criteria for sacroiliitis "highly suggestive of spondyloarthritis (SpA)" required bone marrow edema (BME) seen on a fat-suppressed (FS) sequence, typically short tau inversion recovery or T2-weighted turbo spin echo (T2W), or bone marrow contrast enhancement on a T1-weighted sequence in a typical anatomic area. The lesion must be seen on at least 2 consecutive slices of an MRI scan. The criteria further specify that if there is evidence of inflammation on 1 imaging slice, although with multiple lesions, it still may meet sufficient criteria as highly suggestive of SpA. The group noted that in cases whereby it is difficult to determine whether the lesion meets criteria, other lesions, such as structural lesions (including erosions, sclerosis, fat metaplasia, or ankylosis) or other inflammatory lesions (including synovitis, enthesitis, or capsulitis) should be assessed, although these lesions alone do not meet criteria.[4]

These criteria were specifically designed for classification rather than diagnosis, with the intent of classifying patients with early disease. There are current controversies and questions regarding their use:

1. Should the spine be included in the routine diagnosis and classification of axSpA?
2. Should MRI replace radiographs as the imaging modality of choice in axSpA?
3. What is the prognostic significance of MRI findings? (**Fig. 1**).

SECTION 1: SHOULD SPINE IMAGING BE INCLUDED IN ASSESSMENT IN SPONDYLOARTHRITIS INTERNATIONAL SOCIETY CRITERIA

The 2009 ASAS MRI classification criteria for axSpA define disease by sacroiliitis on MRI. The criteria purposefully did not include spinal changes in the definition, noting that, after data review, the benefit of adding spinal changes to the MRI classification criteria was unclear. However, the spine may be involved in patients with axSpA, both with and without sacroiliac involvement.[5,6] Spinal lesions seen on MRI were defined by the ASAS/OMERACT MRI group as the presence of $\geq$3 inflammatory lesions in the vertebrae on $\geq$2 consecutive slices.[7] In this section, the data regarding spine MRI in axSpA as it pertains to diagnosis and classification is reviewed.

Patterns of active inflammatory spinal findings on MRI in axSpA have been defined as vertebral body inflammatory lesions, and vertebral inflammatory lesions of facet joint and posterior elements (**Fig. 2**).[8] In 2009, a study was done to validate these definitions in a group of 20 patients with ankylosing spondylitis (AS) who had their MRIs scored independently by 4 readers.[9] The study found that, for vertebral corner inflammatory lesions (CILs), interobserver reliability varied substantially, and agreement was less than adequate for most reader pairs (kappa <0.60), although more experienced reader pairs achieved good reliability (kappa >0.68). Lateral segment inflammatory lesions and non-CILs had fair to good reliability among experienced readers (mean

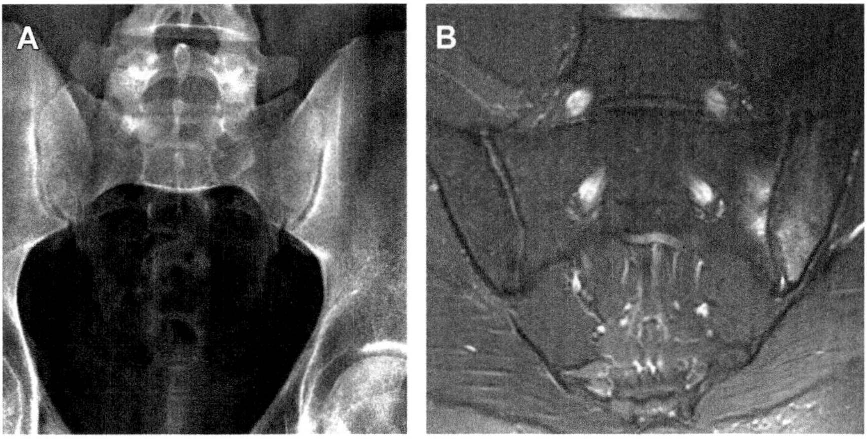

Fig. 1. Pelvic radiograph (*A*) and short tau inversion recovery (STIR) scan (*B*) of a 24-year-old man with an 18-month history of inflammatory type back pain. B27 is positive and CRP is 4 mg/L. Pelvic radiograph is unremarkable. MRI indicates subchondral bone marrow edema in the left iliac and sacral bones meeting the ASAS classification criteria for a positive MRI. The edema is highly suggestive of axSpA because it has a diffuse and extensive distribution in the left iliac and sacral bones, is located in a typical subchondral location, and its appearance is intense in the left sacrum.

kappa = 0.58 and 0.66, respectively). Taken together, these findings suggest that reliability of spinal MRI findings can be quite variable among readers.[9]

The sensitivity and specificity of spinal lesions on MRI for diagnosis of AS has been assessed.[10] In this study, 35 patients with AS, 25 patients with inflammatory back pain (IBP) $\leq$2 years, and 35 healthy controls were evaluated. Spinal inflammatory lesions were defined using the Canada/Denmark International MRI Working Group Criteria as vertebral CILs, non-CILs, and lateral inflammatory lesions. In patients with AS, sensitivity and specificity for $\geq$2 vertebral CILs on MRI were 69% and 94%, respectively, and for patients with IBP, 32% and 96%, respectively. Nine (26%) controls had $\geq$1 CIL, but only 2 (5.7%) controls had greater than 2 CILs. The group concluded that diagnostic usefulness of MRI for AS is optimal when $\geq$2 CILs are present, with a sensitivity and specificity of 69% and 94%, respectively, although the study demonstrated that a single CIL can be found in up to 26% of healthy individuals. These data demonstrate that there is the potential for spinal MRI to have high diagnostic usefulness at a threshold of $\geq$2 CILs given the possible finding of single lesions in healthy individuals. A limitation of this study was that MRI was not evaluated in consecutive patients presenting with undiagnosed back pain. Moreover, MRI assessment was confined to the spine, so that the added value of spine imaging to assessment of the sacroiliac joint (SIJ) alone could not be determined.

The ASAS/OMERACT group later defined spinal involvement in axSpA on MRI as $\geq$3 CILs on $\geq$2 spinal MRI slices. The diagnostic value of this ASAS-OMERACT definition for nr-axSpA and AS was assessed in 2 independent cohorts of patients (A/B) aged $\leq$50 years with undiagnosed back pain referred to outpatient rheumatology clinics.[11] Cohort A comprised 42 patients with back pain referred for further evaluation for suspected axSpA and had 20 healthy age-matched controls, and cohort B comprised 88 patients presenting with acute anterior uveitis with past or present back pain who were referred for assessment of axSpA. The patients were diagnosed based on clinical examination and radiographs as nonradiographic axSpA (nr-axSpA),

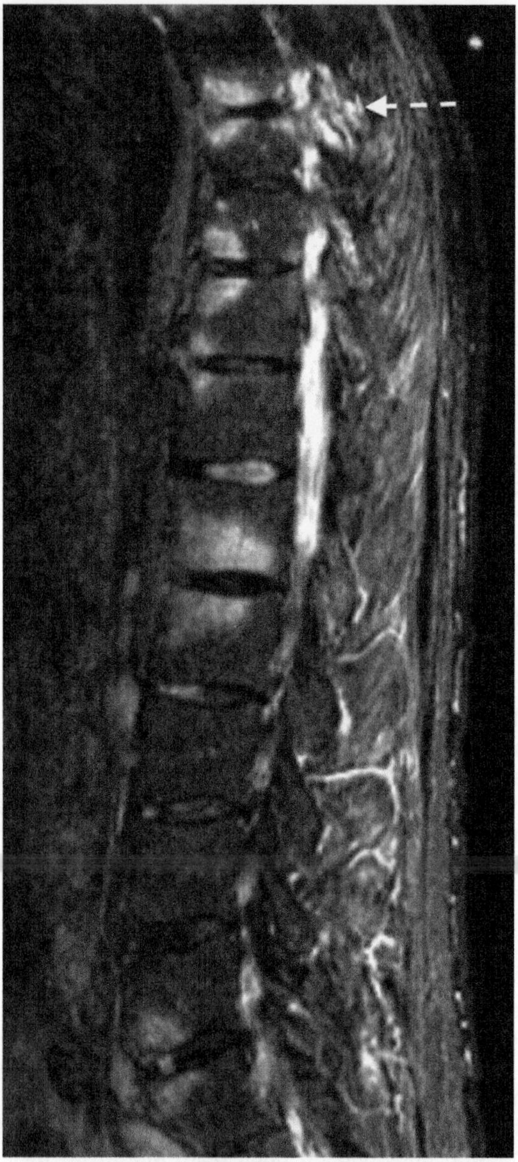

Fig. 2. Short tau inversion recovery (STIR) MRI scan of a 42-year-old man with a history of severe interscapular pain in addition to inflammatory type lower back pain. B27 is positive and CRP is 16 mg/L. There are numerous areas of bone marrow edema at anterior vertebral corners of the lumbar and thoracic spine. There is also facet joint edema in a lateral spinal slice (*dashed arrow*).

AS, or nonspecific back pain (NSBP). Several previously proposed candidate criteria and threshold lesion definitions for spinal MRI in the diagnosis of axSpA were also tested. This study found that neither the ASAS-OMERACT definition nor any other cut-offs for numbers of inflammatory spinal lesions possessed sufficient diagnostic use in differentiating patients with nr-axSpA from NSBP.

The diagnostic value of spine MRI, in addition to SIJ MRI, was studied in the same 2 cohorts (A and B) mentioned in the previous paragraph.[12] The study found that 15% and 24% of patients with nr-axSpA in cohorts A and B, respectively, had negative SIJ MRI and were recategorized as positive for axSpA when combining sacroiliac MRI with spinal MRI. The diagnosis of axSpA improved from low confidence by SIJ MRI to high confidence by combined MRI in 6.6% and 7.3% of patients in cohorts A and B, respectively. However, using SIJ and spinal MRI, 26% (cohort A) and 11% (cohort B) of patients with NSBP and 17.5% of healthy controls with negative SIJ MRI were recategorized as false-positive axSpA. Although the addition of spinal MRI to SIJ MRI identified patients with nr-axSpA not included by SIJ MRI alone, it increased the number of patients incorrectly categorized as nr-axSpA, and the study concluded that combining spine MRI with SIJ MRI added little value to the diagnosis of patients with nr-axSpA. The implication for clinical practice is that considerable caution should be exercised in diagnosing axSpA if there are a limited number of spinal lesions, especially if confined to vertebral corners, and if the MRI of the SIJ appears normal. Both inflammatory and fat lesions may be observed at vertebral corners in patients with degenerative disorders affecting the disc, and even in healthy individuals with no additional abnormalities on imaging of the spine.

To further explore the clinical usefulness of spinal MRI in the diagnosis of axSpA, a study from the SPACE cohort, a group of patients with inflammatory low back pain of ≥3 months but ≤2 years, with onset less than 45 years of age, examined spine and sacroiliac lesions on MRI.[6] Patients were divided into 3 groups: patients with radiographic sacroiliitis, patients without radiographic sacroiliitis but with sacroiliitis on MRI, and patients without sacroiliitis on MRI and radiography. The study found that 51.6% of patients showed BME on MRI of the spine and 56.7% of patients with BME on MRI of the SIJ. Of the patients with BME on MRI spine, 15% had negative sacroiliac MRI and, of the patients without MRI or radiographic evidence of sacroiliitis, 30% had BME spine lesions on MRI. These findings suggest the potential for spinal MRI to identify patients with axSpA that would not have been identified by SIJ MRI alone, although diagnostic usefulness was not formally tested in this study. The study also found that the site of pain correlated significantly with BME lesions in the thoracic and buttock areas, suggesting that spinal imaging could possess greater diagnostic value in the setting of patients with discrete areas of spinal pain. However, a later Dutch study from 2016 investigated spinal imaging findings with regard to localization of pain in patients from the spondyloarthritis caught early (SPACE) cohort and found that spinal pain correlated significantly with imaging findings of degenerative lesions, and that axSpA spinal lesions were not associated with pain.[13]

The frequency of spine lesions on MRI in patients presenting with undiagnosed back pain was examined in a 2015 analysis of the French Cohort of Undifferentiated Spondyloarthritis (DESIR) cohort, a group of French patients with early IBP suggestive of axSpA.[14] The study evaluated the validity of the imaging and clinical arms of the ASAS criteria. Patients who met the ASAS criteria were divided into those fulfilling the imaging criteria, defined as patients with objective signs of SIJ inflammation on MRI or radiographs and at least 1 feature suggestive of SpA, and those fulfilling only the clinical criteria, defined as HLA-B27 positivity with at least 2 features suggestive of axSpA without signs of disease on imaging. Inflammatory changes of the spine on MRI were found in 35.1% and 12.9% of patients in the imaging and clinical arms, respectively. Of the patients in the imaging arm, 38.6% of patients with spinal MRI findings also had SIJ MRI inflammatory changes. Inflammatory spinal lesions on MRI were seen in 21.9% of patients in the clinical arm and with an increased C-reactive protein (CRP). These data again pointed to patients who met clinical criteria for axSpA who did not have sacroiliitis on radiographs or MRI, but were found to have inflammatory spinal disease on MRI, although these numbers were small.

A study using data from the SPACE cohort evaluated various MRI lesions in the spine and SIJ, including inflammation, fatty lesions, erosions, sclerosis/ankylosis, and syndesmophytes.[15] These findings were compared with the imaging and clinical arms of the ASAS axSpA criteria. Whereas MRI spinal lesions were previously defined as the presence of $\geq$3 inflammatory lesions in the vertebrae on $\geq$2 consecutive slices,[7] this study defined a positive MRI by at least 5 lesions according to a specificity cutoff of $\geq$95%. The study reported a positive spine MRI in 18.2% of patients with radiographic disease, defined by the modified New York (mNY) criteria, 21.6% of 2009 ASAS MRI(+) mNY(−) patients, 1.9% of 2009 ASAS clinical-arm patients, 6.7% of possible axSpA patients and 4.3% of no axSpA patients. Similar to the study in the DESIR cohort mentioned above, these data demonstrate that, while spinal MRI did capture patients who otherwise did not have positive imaging findings, overall, the added value of spinal MRI was small.

A study done in 2017 assessed whether it would be advantageous to add MRI spine to the imaging criteria of the ASAS classification criteria by evaluating the prevalence of spinal inflammation in patients from the DESIR and SPACE cohorts.[16] The study examined baseline SIJ radiography and MRI, as well as baseline MRI of the spine. Five hundred and forty-one patients from the SPACE cohort and 650 patients from the DESIR cohort were included in the study. Of these patients, a positive MRI spine was seen in 1% of SPACE and 7% of DESIR patients. Only 1% (SPACE) and 2% (DESIR) of the patients had positive MRI spine without sacroiliitis on imaging, similarly demonstrating that MRI spine adds little to the classification of axSpA.

Currently defined MRI criteria for the classification of axSpA include only SIJ involvement. For diagnosis, there is evidence that patients may also have spinal disease detectable on MRI; however, spinal MRI findings in the absence of radiographic or MRI SIJ findings are uncommon, especially in early disease. In general, spine MRI does not meaningfully contribute to diagnosis or classification and furthermore, specificity may be lost due to false-positive findings at vertebral corners. Currently, the recommendation that classification and routine diagnostic evaluation should be limited to SIJ alone is reasonable. However, in patients suspected of axSpA with equivocal SIJ findings on MRI and radiographs, there may be a role for using spine MRI to assess disease, particularly when the index of clinical suspicion is high and a major treatment decision is pending.

SECTION 2: SHOULD MRI REPLACE RADIOGRAPHS?

Detection and definition of patients with early axSpA, when treatment may be more effective, remains a continuous challenge. Diagnosis is often made years after symptoms develop,[1] when radiographic damage is first noted. Even when radiographs are used to make the diagnosis of axSpA, agreement among readers is only fair to moderate.[17,18] MRI, however, can detect SIJ inflammation at a much earlier time point,[19] which has allowed for the identification of axSpA early in its disease course. In 2009, the ASAS/OMERACT MRI group created classification criteria for axSpA, which, for the first time, included the MRI finding of BME in the SIJ as the criterion lesion.[3,4] In addition, although erosions are not included in the classification criteria, they may be seen in a substantial proportion of patients with nr-axSpA and can be detected on MRI of the SIJ before they are seen on radiography.[20] To aid in early diagnosis and treatment, the European Society of Musculoskeletal Radiology similarly advocated for the use of MRI when axSpA is suspected and radiographs are negative or equivocal.[21]

Given the ability of MRI to detect lesions earlier than radiographs, and the unreliability of radiographic assessment in early disease, is it reasonable to replace radiographic imaging completely with MRI?

Early studies have described the ability of MRI to detect disease before it becomes radiographically apparent. A small prospective study from 1996 evaluated the detection of sacroiliitis by a variety of imaging modalities, including MRI and radiography, in 44 patients with inflammatory low back pain compared with 20 controls. This study found that MRI was more sensitive and specific than radiography in identifying active sacroiliitis and found an additional 75% of cases that were not detected by radiography.[22] A 1999 study examined early development of sacroiliitis on MRI compared with plain radiography.[23] At baseline, 72% of the SIJs studied had sacroiliitis on MRI and, after 3 years, only 47% of SIJs had evidence of sacroiliitis on radiography. These early studies illustrate the ability of MRI to detect sacroiliitis earlier than radiography.

A key question is whether MRI has improved sensitivity and specificity compared with radiography. A study from 2015 examined the histologic features of sacroiliitis and their correlation with imaging findings on MRI, PET-computed tomography (CT), CT, and radiographs in a group of patients considered to have axSpA according to the 2009 ASAS criteria.[24] This study found histologic evidence of sacroiliitis, defined as osteomyelitis, pannus formation, inflammatory cell infiltration, and pathologic changes of the cartilage or subchondral bone, in 81% of patients. MRI demonstrated sacroiliitis in 80.5% of patients, whereas radiography detected these changes in only 52.7% patients. For the detection of sacroiliitis, the study found a sensitivity of 96.4% for MRI and 64.2% for radiographs, with a corresponding specificity of 75% for MRI and 87.5% for radiographs. MRI can identify cartilage involvement, BME, and fat deposition, which improves the sensitivity for early diagnosis of sacroiliitis, and this study demonstrates the superior sensitivity of MRI compared with radiographs for the detection of sacroiliitis.

A study from the same year compared radiography and MRI in the diagnosis of sacroiliitis in patients with chronic back pain $\geq$3 months, aged $\leq$45 years, and referred by a rheumatologist for clinical suspicion of SpA.[25] Radiography and MRI were done to compare these 2 imaging modalities for diagnosing sacroiliitis in patients clinically suspected to have SpA. The study found the sensitivity and specificity of radiography to be 22% and 94%, respectively, while that of MRI was 71% and 90%, respectively. MRI diagnosed sacroiliitis in 39.5% of patients without radiographic changes. To further compare MRI and radiography in the evaluation of axSpA, a 2017 study compared MRI with radiography in detecting structural lesions of the SIJs with low-dose CT as the reference in patients referred to a rheumatologist for possible SpA.[26] This group included patients with axSpA (AS and nr-axSpA) as well as non-SpA. MRI demonstrated significantly better sensitivity for erosion and joint space changes, but lower sensitivity for sclerosis, without a compromise in specificity. For overall positivity for the finding of sacroiliitis the sensitivity of MRI was 85% compared with 48% for radiography without a significant difference in specificity between the 2 imaging modalities, which was greater than 80% for both. These data demonstrate the enhanced sensitivity of MRI compared with radiography in the identification of sacroiliitis, as well as its ability to detect lesions not radiographically apparent.

MRI permits the visualization of inflammation, as well as of structural and bony changes. A challenge in the use of MRI in axSpA pertains to its specificity, as there are numerous other conditions, pathologic as well as physiologic, in which characteristic lesions of axSpA may be seen.[27] A 2010 study investigated the diagnostic usefulness of MRI in differentiating patients with axSpA from patients with IBP and NSBP, and healthy volunteers.[20] SIJ MRIs were done and assessed for BME, fat infiltration, erosion, and anklyosis. The study found that ASAS-defined BME was evident in 85.3% of patients with AS, 66.7% of patients with IBP, 23.1% of patients with NSBP, and 6.8% of healthy controls. A single BME lesion was seen in 26.9% of the patients with NSBP and in 22% of the healthy control subjects. This study illustrates that MRI findings consistent with BME can be seen in patients without axSpA and can contribute to false-positive results (**Fig. 3**).

A cross-sectional analysis carried out in 2016 corroborated similar challenges with the application of MRI in the identification of axSpA. This study assessed MRI scans from the Spines of Southern Denmark Center, a referral center for non-IBP and estimated the prevalence ASAS criteria MRI findings and clinical features for axSpA in patients ≤40 years old with low pretest probability for axSpA.[28] While 21% of patients from this population demonstrated active sacroiliitis according to the ASAS definition, it previously had been shown that only 5% of unselected patients with chronic low back pain had spondyloarthritis (AS and undifferentiated SpA).[29–31] Similarly, a study using National Health and Nutrition Examination Survey data demonstrated the prevalence of axSpA and AS to be 1.4% and 0.55%, respectively.[32] The study illustrates that a positive MRI defined by ASAS criteria should not be used to diagnose axSpA in an unselected population of young patients with chronic low back pain as it has the potential to incorrectly identify several patients as axSpA who do not have this disease.

To further demonstrate the challenge of specificity in MRI, a study investigated SIJ MRI in patients with axSpA compared with patients with mechanical back pain syndromes and healthy controls from the SPACE cohort.[33] The study included patients with axSpA, women with postpartum back pain, patients with chronic back pain, and healthy subjects (including frequent runners). The study found that 91.5% of patients with axSpA, 57.1% of patients with postpartum back pain, 23.4% of healthy volunteers, 12.5% of runners, and 6.4% of patients with chronic back pain had sacroiliitis on MRI defined by the ASAS classification criteria and Spondyloarthritis Research Consortium of Canada scoring index. However, "deep" BME lesions, defined as lesions ≥1 cm from the articular surface, were not found in healthy volunteers, patients with chronic back pain, or runners, although these findings were found in axSpA and

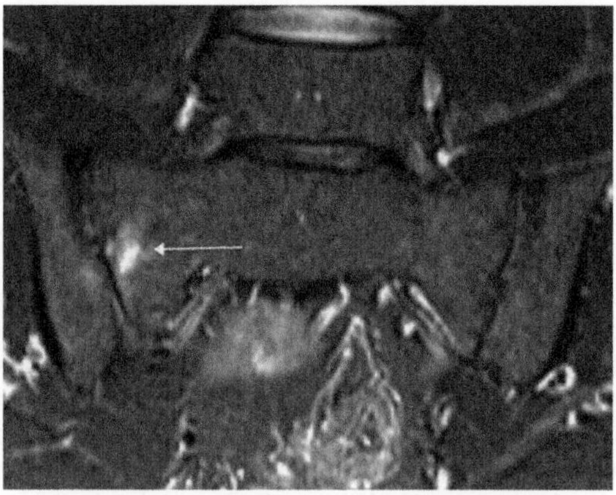

Fig. 3. Short tau inversion recovery (STIR) MRI scan of a 39-year-old man with a 3-year history of lower back pain with inflammatory characteristics but B27 is negative and CRP is 3.7 mg/L. There is a small focal area of bone marrow edema in the right sacrum (*arrow*). This may be seen in the early stages of osteoarthritis and is false-positive for axSpA.

patients with postpartum back pain. A recent article evaluated the frequency of SIJ MRI features in the SIJs of athletes.[34] The study assessed SIJ MRI in recreational runners and ice hockey players for BME and structural lesions to identify patients who met the ASAS definition of active sacroiliitis and might have false-positive structural lesions. The study found that 30% to 35% of runners and 41% of hockey players fulfilled the ASAS definition of active sacroiliitis. These studies demonstrate that typical inflammatory lesions on MRI can be seen in groups of patients without clinical axSpA. Conversely, erosion and fat metaplasia were much less frequent and therefore more specific for axSpA.

Although MRI has been shown to be more sensitive than radiography in identifying sacroiliitis, the challenge of false-positives remains. A study done in 2015 sought to identify a method to improve the specificity of MRI in identifying axSpA by developing candidate lesion-based criteria.[35] This study was done in 2 cohorts of patients (A/B), described in the previous section, who developed back pain at age $\leq$50 presenting for assessment of axSpA. Patients were classified according to the rheumatologists's expert opinion based on clinical examination, radiography, and laboratories as nr-axSpA, AS, or NSBP. SIJ MRI were assessed by 4 blinded readers by global evaluation followed by BME/erosions assessment in each SIJ quadrant. From this examination, candidate lesion-based criteria were created based on the number of SIJ quadrants. In evaluating the sensitivity and specificity of candidate criteria for nr-axSpA versus NSBP, the study found that for cohorts A/B, global assessment showed high specificity (95%/83%) compared with the ASAS definition (76%/74%). However, BME $\geq$3 SIJ quadrants (89%/84%) or $\geq$4 SIJ quadrants (92%/87%) demonstrated high specificity compared with both global assessment and the ASAS definition. The study found that erosions in $\geq$2 SIJ quadrants and/or BME in $\geq$3 SIJ quadrants had a sensitivity of 83%/46%, comparably high with global assessment (74%/44%) and the ASAS defenition (sensitivity 80%/42%), while the specificity for erosion in $\geq$2 SIJ quadrants and/or BME of $\geq$3 SIJ quadrants (85%/82%) was not affected compared with the specificity of the ASAS criteria. This study demonstrates that candidate lesion-based criteria can improve the sensitivity without reducing specificity of MRI in the diagnosis of patients with axSpA.

To assess the impact of replacing radiographs with structural lesions on MRI in the classification of axSpA, a study using the DESIR cohort examined the use of MRI compared with radiographs in classification of axSpA.[19] One aim of the study was to evaluate the usefulness of replacing radiographic sacroiliitis with MRI in evaluating SIJ structural lesions (MRI-SI-s) with regard to the performance of the imaging arm of the ASAS classification criteria. Although the study evaluated structural, noncriteria lesions, it found that, when MRI-SI-s replaced radiographs, classification did not change in most patients and, if it did, it was generally within subgroups of the criteria. A small number of patients (1%–2%), however, were no longer classified with axSpA. The authors concluded that structural lesions on MRI can be used reliably either as an addition to, or as a substitute for, radiographs in the classification of axSpA. MRI may help ameliorate the burden of radiation exposure, although the authors noted the issue of cost, availability, and caution in interpretation, as they found MRI-SI-s agreement among radiologists to be only moderate. For these reasons, the authors conclude that MRI-SI-s can provide adjunctive information to ASAS axSpA classification criteria but do not recommend the replacement of radiographs with MRI-SI-s.

A study using the SPACE cohort similarly investigated the usefulness of replacing radiographic sacroiliitis with MRI-SI-s in the classification of axSpA by ASAS criteria.[36] When MRI-SI-s was used instead of radiographs, classification did not change in 97.3% of patients. One percent of unclassified patients would be classified as axSpA, although 1.7% would not be classified as axSpA. The group concluded that using MRI-SI-s instead of conventional radiographs did not change ASAS axSpA classification in most patients with early disease. However, the group advocated for the addition of MRI-SI-s rather than replacement of radiographs in the ASAS axSpA criteria, citing challenges such as cost, accessibility, and familiarity with the radiographic mNY criteria compared with MRI-SI-s interpretation.

It has been shown that, when radiographs are used in the classification of SpA, agreement among readers is only fair to moderate.[18] Magnetic resonance imaging, however, has demonstrated appropriate inter-reader reliability in axSpA. A study using the DESIR cohort compared baseline MRI SIJ readings by local radiologists/rheumatologists to centrally trained readers experienced in scoring SIJ MRI.[37] The study found good inter-reader agreement between 2 central readers (k = 0.73) and between central and local readers (k = 0.70). The study found disagreement between local and central readers in 13.4% of MRI SIJ; however, in patients with IBP, classification of only 7.9% of patients changed based on a different evaluator's assessment of images. These data demonstrate the degree of reliability of the MRI criteria compared with radiography in the identification of axSpA.

In axSpA, MRI detects lesions not seen radiographically without the risk of radiation exposure, allowing for early identification of disease and prompt initiation of treatment. This is particularly important in a population that is likely to undergo a significant amount of imaging. However, issues regarding the availability and cost of MRI, the specificity of ASAS-defined sacroiliitis on MRI, as well as reliability in interpretation, remain a challenge in advocating for replacing radiographs completely. Although MRI is a very sensitive imaging modality, and particularly helpful in evaluating patients with early axSpA, it also detects findings consistent with sacroiliitis in patients without axSpA. Currently, the 2015 European League Against Rheumatism recommendations support conventional radiography of the SIJ in diagnosing axSpA and the use of SIJ MRI to evaluate for inflammatory or structural lesions as an alternative first-imaging method or if diagnosis cannot be otherwise established.[38] Although MRI has been found to be reliably sensitive, MRI findings should be interpreted in the appropriate clinical context and not used in isolation, particularly in patients in whom the diagnosis of axSpA is less likely.

SECTION 3: DO MRI CHANGES HAVE PROGNOSTIC SIGNIFICANCE?

It is well established that radiographic changes have prognostic significance, although radiographic progression of disease is slow. This was demonstrated in a study characterizing radiographic changes in the spine in a group of patients with AS followed prospectively for a mean 7.9 years.[39] The study found that 72% of patients demonstrated radiographic progression of disease, although 24% of patients did not. HLA-B27 positivity, male gender, and more severe baseline Stoke AS Spine Score, a score that qualifies structural changes on radiographs at the vertebral corners, were associated with more rapid radiographic progression of disease. In axSpA, CRP has also been shown to be associated with radiographic progression of disease.[40]

Given the prognostic role of radiography in axSpA, an important clinical question is whether MRI predicts progression of disease in axSpA. A 1999 article evaluated the prognostic value of MRI in 25 patients with inflammatory low back pain and radiographic sacroiliitis grade $\leq$2 using the mNY criteria. At baseline, about 72% of the total SIJs had abnormalities on MRI. After 3 years of follow-up, 48% of patients developed grade $\geq$2 sacroiliitis on radiography, suggesting that inflammation observed on MRI may predict radiographic progression of disease.[23,41]

The prognostic role of MRI was evaluated in a 2008 study that investigated the progression from MRI sacroiliitis to AS, diagnosed radiographically by mNY criteria, at 8 years in a group of undiagnosed patients with early IBP (<2 years). At baseline, 83% of patients had MRI-evident sacroiliitis, and at follow-up 33.3% progressed to AS. The study found that severe sacroiliitis seen on MRI and HLA-B27 positivity were excellent predictors of future AS, while mild or no sacroiliitis, independent of HLA-B27 status, was a predictor of not progressing to AS.[42] The combination of severe sacroiliitis seen on MRI and HLA-B27 positivity was associated with a likelihood ratio of 8 for development of future AS, while mild or with no sacroiliitis, regardless of HLA-B27 status, was a predictor of not having AS (likelihood ratio of 0.3). This study illustrates that MRI findings correlate with progression of disease.

The relationship between inflammation and new bone formation has been, and remains, challenging to define. One study evaluated spinal MRI and radiographs in a group of patients with AS treated with antitumor necrosis factor (anti-TNF) therapy and compared baseline MRI inflammation with the development of vertebral syndesmophytes at 2 years.[43] The study found that new bone formation occurred more frequently in areas with spinal inflammation on baseline MRI than in those without. However, there was evidence of new bone formation in areas without inflammation at baseline, suggesting both a relationship between inflammation and syndesmophyte formation and some uncoupling of this process.

A group of studies further evaluated the relationship between axial inflammation on MRI and the development of radiographic change. One study followed patients treated with anti-TNF agents for 2 years and investigated whether an active inflammatory lesion on MRI was more likely to evolve into a syndesmophyte on radiography.[44] This study found that syndesmophytes developed significantly more frequently in vertebral corners with inflammation on baseline MRI. A 2011 study evaluated whether vertebral CILs on MRI were more likely to develop into radiographic syndesmophytes compared with a vertebral corner without a CIL over a mean of 19.2 months.[45] The study found that new syndesmophytes developed significantly more frequently from vertebral corners where a CIL had completely resolved on MRI compared with vertebral corners without CILs in patients treated with anti-TNF therapy. These data suggest a relationship between the resolution of inflammation and the development of new bone.

A long-term study that evaluated the progression of lesions on MRI examined a group of patients with axSpA over 2 to 7 years to assess the prognostic significance of subchondral edema, erosions, and fatty marrow deposition on MRI of the SIJ. Lesions were scored via the Danish scoring method, which evaluates and grades features at multiple osseous and joint space positions.[46] The study found that MRI scores for chronic SIJ changes significantly increased over this period, most strikingly in patients who were HLA-B27-positive and in patients fulfilling the mNY criteria for AS. SIJ activity scores $\geq$2, erosion scores $\geq$1, and fatty marrow deposition scores $\geq$4 at baseline were significantly related to progression of chronic SIJ changes. SIJ activity or chronic changes on MRI at baseline were related to progression of chronic changes and the presence of AS according to mNY criteria, demonstrating that inflammatory and chronic lesions seen on MRI predict progression to AS.

Various studies have demonstrated that chronic lesions on MRI develop from areas of inflammation. A 2011 study prospectively evaluated the relationship between active inflammatory lesions on MRI and the development of chronic lesions of the spine and SIJ on whole body MRI over 1 year.[47] The study examined patients enrolled in the etanercept versus sulfasalazine in early axial spondyloarthritis on active inflammatory lesions as detected by whole-body MRI (ESTHER) trial, a prospective randomized control trial of etanercept versus sulfasalazine for 48 weeks in patients with axSpA. The study found a significant relationship between the resolution of inflammation and the development of fatty lesions in the SIJ. Another study examined the connection between focal fat lesions at vertebral corners and the development of new syndesmophytes on MRI in patients with AS in 2 cohorts of patients, a clinical trial cohort of anti-TNF therapy compared with placebo, and an observational cohort of patients on standard therapy compared with anti-TNF therapy.[48] The study found that in both cohorts there was significantly more syndesmophyte formation in vertebral corners with fat lesions compared with those without these findings on baseline MRI, supporting the model that chronic changes evolve from inflammatory lesions.

Long-term studies have explored the relationship between early changes seen on MRI and the development of radiographic disease. A study from 2012 examined the usefulness of needle biopsy in the diagnosis of early sacroiliitis and included imaging data.[49] In this study, all patients underwent needle biopsy of the SIJ, and MRI was used to confirm the presence or absence of sacroiliitis in a subset of the patients. The study found that, after 5 to 10 years of follow-up, 87.5% of patients with MRI sacroiliitis at baseline developed radiographic evidence of sacroiliitis, although 30% of patients without sacroiliitis on MRI at baseline also developed radiographic disease. Another long-term study investigated the validity of the 2009 ASAS classification criteria and examined how baseline ASAS-defined MRI findings correlate with radiographic progression at 8 years in patients with early IBP.[50] When excluding patients with baseline radiographic sacroiliitis, the study found 47.6% of patients had an increase in radiographic sacroiliitis at 8 years, and 90% of these patients had an abnormal baseline MRI. The study found that subjects who developed AS tended to have a significantly greater number of SIJ quadrants with BME at baseline, and patients with radiographic AS had significantly higher scores of BME at baseline compared with patients who did not. However, 39% of patients with $\geq$5 SIJ quadrants with BME and 33.3% patients who had $\geq$10 SIJ quadrants with BME had mild or no radiographic progression at follow-up with only a small minority receiving disease-modifying antirheumatic drug therapy. Taken together, these data demonstrated that there is an inconsistent relationship between MRI findings of inflammation and prognosis for radiographic disease.

Further evidence suggesting a weak relationship between MRI findings and progression of disease was demonstrated in a study using a random sample of patients from the Asymptomatic Atrial Fibrillation and Stroke Evaluation in Pacemaker Patients and the Ankylosing Spondylitis Study for the Evaluation of Recombinant Infliximab Therapy (ASSERT) database, a 24-week randomized control trial of infliximab in patients with active AS. This study evaluated the relationship between MRI inflammation in the spine and the formation of syndesmophytes.[51] This study found that inflammation on MRI slightly increased the tendency to form a new syndesmophyte but did not predict the growth of already existing syndesmophytes. The study found that most new syndesmophytes developed in vertebral units without inflammation, similarly demonstrating a weak link between inflammation seen on MRI and the development of new bone formation.

Conversely, other data have demonstrated a more nuanced relationship between MRI inflammation and the formation of new bone. A study evaluating adalimumab in AS assessed whether new bone formation developed from acute inflammation or advanced inflammatory lesions.[52] The study distinguished between acute inflammatory lesions and advanced vertebral CILs, characterized as chronic lesions demonstrating fat infiltration, sclerosis, or erosion on MRI. The study found that new syndesmophytes developed from advanced vertebral CILs significantly more frequently than from locations with acute or no vertebral CILs. These findings support the notion that new bone formation develops from advanced inflammatory lesions, evolving more predictably from fat metaplasia. Similarly, in another study, SIJ MRIs were assessed at baseline and after 2 years in patients from the Follow Up Research Cohort in Ankylosing Spondylitis.[53] The study found that reduction in erosions and increase in fat metaplasia were independently associated with the development of new ankylosis.

The use of MRI as a tool in predicting radiographic progression was demonstrated in further studies. A study from 2014 evaluated the relationship between spinal inflammation and fat metaplasia on MRI and radiographic new bone formation in AS.[54] Radiographs and spinal MRIs were done at baseline, and at 2 and 5 years, in patients with AS. Vertebral edges with inflammation and fat metaplasia at baseline had the highest risk for syndesmophyte formation at 5 years. A study from 2016 studied the relationship between inflammatory lesions seen on MRI and development of radiographic syndesmophytes.[55] The study reviewed spinal MRIs at baseline, and at 24 and 102 weeks, from patients in the ASSERT study. The study found that vertebral corner inflammation and vertebral fat deposition were associated with new bone formation in AS. Given the characteristic evolution of lesions seen on MRI in these studies, these data highlight the capacity for MRI to be used prognostically.

The relationship between MRI findings and radiographic progression of disease was studied in the DESIR cohort. This study investigated the rate of progression of radiographic sacroiliitis over 2 years.[56] This study analyzed the percentage of patients classified as nr-axSpA at baseline who developed radiographic axSpA after 2 years. Sixty-six percent of patients with baseline positive radiographs had MRI SIJ inflammation at baseline, while 26.4% of patients with baseline-negative radiographs had positive MRI SIJ at baseline. The percentage of patients who progressed from nr-axSpA to radiographic axSpA was 17.3% for patients with baseline MRI SIJ inflammation versus 0% of patients without baseline MRI SIJ inflammation. Baseline MRI SIJ inflammation was an independent predictor of meeting the radiographic mNY criteria, with an odds ratio (OR) of 48.8, demonstrating the prognostic significance of MRI. The study found that smoking (OR = 12.6) and HLA B27 positivity (12.6) were similarly independent predictors of progression from nr-axSpA to axSpA. Interestingly, CRP was not shown to correlate with radiographic progression.

A 5-year follow-up of this study evaluated SIJ radiographic progression and its relation to MRI inflammation.[57] SIJ radiographs and MRI were evaluated at baseline, and at 2 and 5 years, in patients with new onset axSpA from the DESIR cohort. Progression was defined as progression from nr-axSpA to radiographic sacroiliitis or change in at least 1 grade of disease. The study found that radiographic progression occurred in 5% to 13% of patients and baseline MRI SIJ predicted structural damage after 5 years in both B27-positive and B27-negative patients exhibiting the potential for MRI to be used as a prognostic indicator for radiographic progression of disease. At the 5-year follow-up, neither smoking nor B27 status was predictive of radiographic progression.

There is an increasing body of literature supporting MRI as a prognostic tool in predicting radiographic progression of disease and the development of AS. However, the evolution of these changes remains unclear. There is evidence that inflammatory lesions develop predictably into new bone formation; however, a dissociation of this process has also been demonstrated, with new bone formation arising from areas without inflammation. Given the potential for inflammatory lesions to progress to radiographic disease, the detection of early inflammation on MRI may provide a window of opportunity for disease modification before the development of permanent damage.[52] The challenge is identifying the patients at risk, the time frame for the development of these lesions and the specific MRI lesions that are predictive of radiographic changes.

MRI provides an important imaging tool to assess axSpA, particularly early in the disease course, before radiographic damage is apparent. For this reason, MRI was incorporated into the 2009 ASAS/OMERACT classification criteria for axSpA. However, as it is a relatively new imaging modality, challenges remain. Future directions to address these challenges include a need to refine MRI techniques to improve the specificity of MRI to reduce the number of false-positive reports and "background noise," as well as the development of more accurate definitions of a positive MRI. To better understand disease evolution and guide treatment decisions, the pathophysiologic relationship between inflammation and chronic damage and the role of MRI in monitoring disease progression should be evaluated further.

REFERENCES

1. Feldtkeller E, Khan MA, van der Heijde D, et al. Age at disease onset and diagnosis delay in HLA-B27 negative vs. positive patients with ankylosing spondylitis. Rheumatol Int 2003;23(2):61–6.
2. Maksymowych WP, Wichuk S, Dougados M, et al. MRI evidence of structural changes in the sacroiliac joints of patients with non-radiographic axial spondyloarthritis even in the absence of MRI inflammation. Arthritis Res Ther 2017;19(1):126.
3. Rudwaleit M, Jurik AG, Hermann KG, et al. Defining active sacroiliitis on magnetic resonance imaging (MRI) for classification of axial spondyloarthritis: a consensual approach by the ASAS/OMERACT MRI group. Ann Rheum Dis 2009;68(10):1520–7.
4. Lambert RG, Bakker PA, van der Heijde D, et al. Defining active sacroiliitis on MRI for classification of axial spondyloarthritis: update by the ASAS MRI working group. Ann Rheum Dis 2016;75(11):1958–63.
5. van der Heijde D, Sieper J, Maksymowych WP, et al. Spinal inflammation in the absence of sacroiliac joint inflammation on magnetic resonance imaging in patients with active nonradiographic axial spondyloarthritis. Arthritis Rheumatol 2014;66(3):667–73.
6. Lorenzin M, Ortolan A, Frallonardo P, et al. Spine and sacroiliac joints on magnetic resonance imaging in patients with early axial spondyloarthritis: prevalence of lesions and association with clinical and disease activity indices from the Italian group of the SPACE study. Reumatismo 2016;68(2):72–82.
7. Hermann KG, Baraliakos X, van der Heijde DM, et al. Descriptions of spinal MRI lesions and definition of a positive MRI of the spine in axial spondyloarthritis: a consensual approach by the ASAS/OMERACT MRI study group. Ann Rheum Dis 2012;71(8):1278–88.
8. Lambert RG, Pedersen SJ, Maksymowych WP, et al. Active inflammatory lesions detected by magnetic resonance imaging in the spine of patients with spondyloarthritis – definitions, assessment system, and reference image set. J Rheumatol Suppl 2009;(84):3–17.
9. Pededrsen SJ, Østergaard M, Chiowchanwisawakit P, et al. Validation of definitions for active inflammatory lesions detected by magnetic resonance imaging in the spine of patients with spondyloarthritis. J Rheumatol 2009;84:35–8.
10. Weber U, Hodler J, Kubik RA, et al. Sensitivity and specificity of spinal inflammatory lesions assessed by whole-body magnetic resonance imaging in patients

with ankylosing spondylitis or recent-onset inflammatory back pain. Arthritis Rheum 2009;61(7):900–8.
11. Weber U, Zhao Z, Rufibach K, et al. Diagnostic utility of candidate definitions for demonstrating axial spondyloarthritis on magnetic resonance imaging of the spine. Arthritis Rheumatol 2015;67(4):924–33.
12. Weber U, Zubler V, Zhao Z, et al. Does spinal MRI add incremental diagnostic value to MRI of the sacroiliac joints alone in patients with non-radiographic axial spondyloarthritis? Ann Rheum Dis 2015;74(6):985–92.
13. de Hooge M, de Bruin F, de Beer L, et al. Is the site of back pain related to the location of magnetic resonance imaging lesions in patients with chronic back pain? results from the spondyloarthritis caught early cohort. Arthritis Care Res (Hoboken) 2017;69(5):717–23.
14. Molto A, Paternotte S, van der Heijde D, et al. Evaluation of the validity of the different arms of the ASAS set of criteria for axial spondyloarthritis and description of the different imaging abnormalities suggestive of spondyloarthritis: data from the DESIR cohort. Ann Rheum Dis 2015;74(4):746–51.
15. de Hooge M, van den Berg R, Navarro-Compan V, et al. Patients with chronic back pain of short duration from the SPACE cohort: which MRI structural lesions in the sacroiliac joints and inflammatory and structural lesions in the spine are most specific for axial spondyloarthritis? Ann Rheum Dis 2016;75(7):1308–14.
16. Ez-Zaitouni Z, Bakker PA, van Lunteren M, et al. The yield of a positive MRI of the spine as imaging criterion in the ASAS classification criteria for axial spondyloarthritis: results from the SPACE and DESIR cohorts. Ann Rheum Dis 2017;76(10): 1731–6.
17. van den Berg R, Lenczner G, Feydy A, et al. Agreement between clinical practice and trained central reading in reading of sacroiliac joints on plain pelvic radiographs. Results from the DESIR cohort. Arthritis Rheumatol 2014;66(9):2403–11.
18. Christiansen AA, Hendricks O, Kuettel D, et al. Limited reliability of radiographic assessment of sacroiliac joints in patients with suspected early spondyloarthritis. J Rheumatol 2017;44(1):70–7.
19. Bakker PA, van den Berg R, Lenczner G, et al. Can we use structural lesions seen on MRI of the sacroiliac joints reliably for the classification of patients according to the ASAS axial spondyloarthritis criteria? data from the DESIR cohort. Ann Rheum Dis 2017;76(2):392–8.
20. Weber U, Lambert RG, Ostergaard M, et al. The diagnostic utility of magnetic resonance imaging in spondylarthritis: an international multicenter evaluation of one hundred eighty-seven subjects. Arthritis Rheum 2010;62(10):3048–58.
21. Schueller-Weidekamm C, Mascarenhas VV, Sudol-Szopinska I, et al. Imaging and interpretation of axial spondylarthritis: the radiologist's perspective–consensus of the Arthritis Subcommittee of the ESSR. Semin Musculoskelet Radiol 2014;18(3): 265–79.
22. Blum U, Buitrago-Tellez C, Mundinger A, et al. Magnetic resonance imaging (MRI) for detection of active sacroiliitis–a prospective study comparing conventional radiography, scintigraphy, and contrast enhanced MRI. J Rheumatol 1996;23(12):2107–15.
23. Oostveen J, Prevo R, den Boer J, et al. Early detection of sacroiliitis on magnetic resonance imaging and subsequent development of sacroiliitis on plain radiography. A prospective, longitudinal study. J Rheumatol 1999;26(9):1953–8.
24. Cui Y, Zhang X, Zhao Z, et al. The relationship between histopathological and imaging features of sacroiliitis. Int J Clin Exp Med 2015;8(4):5904–10.

25. Sudol-Szopinska I, Kwiatkowska B, Wlodkowska-Korytkowska M, et al. Diagnostics of sacroiliitis according to ASAS criteria: a comparative evaluation of conventional radiographs and MRI in patients with a clinical suspicion of spondyloarthropathy. preliminary results. Pol J Radiol 2015;80:266–76.
26. Diekhoff T, Hermann KG, Greese J, et al. Comparison of MRI with radiography for detecting structural lesions of the sacroiliac joint using CT as standard of reference: results from the SIMACT study. Ann Rheum Dis 2017;76(9):1502–8.
27. Weber U, Maksymowych WP. Sensitivity and specificity of magnetic resonance imaging for axial spondyloarthritis. Am J Med Sci 2011;341(4):272–7.
28. Arnbak B, Grethe Jurik A, Hørslev-Petersen K, et al. Associations between spondyloarthritis features and magnetic resonance imaging findings: a cross-sectional analysis of 1,020 patients with persistent low back pain. Arthritis Rheumatol 2016;68(4):892–900.
29. Underwood MR, Dawes P. Inflammatory back pain in primary care. Br J Rheumatol 1995;34(11):1074–7.
30. Rudwaleit M, van der Heijde D, Khan MA, et al. How to diagnose axial spondyloarthritis early. Ann Rheum Dis 2004;63(5):535–43.
31. Deodhar A. Sacroiliac joint magnetic resonance imaging in the diagnosis of axial spondyloarthritis: "a tiny bit of white on two consecutive slices" may be objective, but not specific. Arthritis Rheumatol 2016;68(4):775–8.
32. Reveille JD, Weisman MH. The epidemiology of back pain, axial spondyloarthritis and HLA-B27 in the United States. Am J Med Sci 2013;345(6):431–6.
33. de Winter J, de Hooge M, van de Sande M, et al. Magnetic resonance imaging of the sacroiliac joints indicating sacroiliitis according to the assessment of spondyloarthritis international society definition in healthy individuals, runners, and women with postpartum back pain. Arthritis Rheumatol 2018;70(7):1042–8.
34. Weber U, Jurik AG, Zejden A, et al. Frequency and anatomic distribution of magnetic resonance imaging features in the sacroiliac joints of young athletes: exploring "background noise" toward a data-driven definition of sacroiliitis in early spondyloarthritis. Arthritis Rheumatol 2018;70(5):736–45.
35. Weber U, Ostergaard M, Lambert RG, et al. Candidate lesion-based criteria for defining a positive sacroiliac joint MRI in two cohorts of patients with axial spondyloarthritis. Ann Rheum Dis 2015;74(11):1976–82.
36. Bakker PA, van den Berg R, Hooge M, et al. Impact of replacing radiographic sacroiliitis by magnetic resonance imaging structural lesions on the classification of patients with axial spondyloarthritis. Rheumatology (Oxford) 2018. https://doi.org/10.1093/rheumatology/kex532.
37. van den Berg R, Lenczner G, Thevenin F, et al. Classification of axial SpA based on positive imaging (radiographs and/or MRI of the sacroiliac joints) by local rheumatologists or radiologists versus central trained readers in the DESIR cohort. Ann Rheum Dis 2015;74(11):2016–21.
38. Mandl P, Navarro-Compan V, Terslev L, et al. EULAR recommendations for the use of imaging in the diagnosis and management of spondyloarthritis in clinical practice. Ann Rheum Dis 2015;74(7):1327–39.
39. Ramiro S, Stolwijk C, van Tubergen A, et al. Evolution of radiographic damage in ankylosing spondylitis: a 12 year prospective follow-up of the OASIS study. Ann Rheum Dis 2015;74(1):52–9.
40. Poddubnyy D, Rudwaleit M, Haibel H, et al. Rates and predictors of radiographic sacroiliitis progression over 2 years in patients with axial spondyloarthritis. Ann Rheum Dis 2011;70(8):1369–74.

41. Maksymowych WP. MRI and X-ray in axial spondyloarthritis: the relationship between inflammatory and structural changes. Arthritis Res Ther 2012;14(2):207.
42. Bennett AN, McGonagle D, O'Connor P, et al. Severity of baseline magnetic resonance imaging-evident sacroiliitis and HLA-B27 status in early inflammatory back pain predict radiographically evident ankylosing spondylitis at eight years. Arthritis Rheum 2008;58(11):3413–8.
43. Baraliakos X, Listing J, Rudwaleit M, et al. The relationship between inflammation and new bone formation in patients with ankylosing spondylitis. Arthritis Res Ther 2008;10(5):R104.
44. Maksymowych WP, Chiowchanwisawakit P, Clare T, et al. Inflammatory lesions of the spine on magnetic resonance imaging predict the development of new syndesmophytes in ankylosing spondylitis: evidence of a relationship between inflammation and new bone formation. Arthritis Rheum 2009;60(1):93–102.
45. Pedersen SJ, Chiowchanwisawakit P, Lambert RG, et al. Resolution of inflammation following treatment of ankylosing spondylitis is associated with new bone formation. J Rheumatol 2011;38(7):1349–54.
46. Madsen KB, Schiottz-Christensen B, Jurik AG. Prognostic significance of magnetic resonance imaging changes of the sacroiliac joints in spondyloarthritis – A Followup Study. J Rheumatol 2010;37(8):1718–27.
47. Song IH, Hermann KG, Haibel H, et al. Relationship between active inflammatory lesions in the spine and sacroiliac joints and new development of chronic lesions on whole-body MRI in early axial spondyloarthritis: results of the ESTHER trial at week 48. Ann Rheum Dis 2011;70(7):1257–63.
48. Chiowchanwisawakit P, Lambert RG, Conner-Spady B, et al. Focal fat lesions at vertebral corners on magnetic resonance imaging predict the development of new syndesmophytes in ankylosing spondylitis. Arthritis Rheum 2011;63(8):2215–25.
49. Gong Y, Zheng N, Chen SB, et al. Ten years' experience with needle biopsy in the early diagnosis of sacroiliitis. Arthritis Rheum 2012;64(5):1399–406.
50. Aydin SZ, Maksymowych WP, Bennett AN, et al. Validation of the ASAS criteria and definition of a positive MRI of the sacroiliac joint in an inception cohort of axial spondyloarthritis followed up for 8 years. Ann Rheum Dis 2012;71(1):56–60.
51. van der Heijde D, Machado P, Braun J, et al. MRI inflammation at the vertebral unit only marginally predicts new syndesmophyte formation: a multilevel analysis in patients with ankylosing spondylitis. Ann Rheum Dis 2012;71(3):369–73.
52. Maksymowych WP, Morency N, Conner-Spady B, et al. Suppression of inflammation and effects on new bone formation in ankylosing spondylitis: evidence for a window of opportunity in disease modification. Ann Rheum Dis 2013;72(1):23–8.
53. Maksymowych WP, Wichuk S, Chiowchanwisawakit P, et al. Fat metaplasia and backfill are key intermediaries in the development of sacroiliac joint ankylosis in patients with ankylosing spondylitis. Arthritis Rheumatol 2014;66(11):2958–67.
54. Baraliakos X, Heldmann F, Callhoff J, et al. Which spinal lesions are associated with new bone formation in patients with ankylosing spondylitis treated with anti-TNF agents? A long-term observational study using MRI and conventional radiography. Ann Rheum Dis 2014;73(10):1819–25.
55. Machado PM, Baraliakos X, van der Heijde D, et al. MRI vertebral corner inflammation followed by fat deposition is the strongest contributor to the development of new bone at the same vertebral corner: a multilevel longitudinal analysis in patients with ankylosing spondylitis. Ann Rheum Dis 2016;75(8):1486–93.

56. Dougados M, Demattei C, van den Berg R, et al. Rate and predisposing factors for sacroiliac joint radiographic progression after a two-year follow-up period in recent-onset spondyloarthritis. Arthritis Rheumatol 2016;68(8):1904–13.
57. Dougados M, Sepriano A, Molto A, et al. Sacroiliac radiographic progression in recent onset axial spondyloarthritis: the 5-year data of the DESIR cohort. Ann Rheum Dis 2017;76(11):1823–8.

Are the Current Recommendations for Chloroquine and Hydroxychloroquine Screening Appropriate?

Sergio Schwartzman, MD[a,*], C. Michael Samson, MD, MBA[b]

KEYWORDS

• Antimalarials • Hydroxychloroquine • Quinacrine • Ocular toxicity • Retinopathy

KEY POINTS

- Hydroxychloroquine and quinacrine are frequently used to treat rheumatic diseases.
- Ocular toxicity, although infrequent, is one of the potential side effects of antimalarial therapies.
- Current recommendations are unifocal in being developed by only ophthalmologists who do not treat patients for their rheumatic diseases.
- The data used to create the recommendations are meager and retrospective.
- Comanagement of patients with rheumatic disease who are exposed to antimalarial therapies requires a greater interaction between ophthalmologists and rheumatologists.

Antimalarial medications, primarily hydroxychloroquine, have become a cornerstone of treatment of chronic rheumatic diseases. Chloroquine is used uncommonly in the United States because it may have an increased incidence of gastrointestinal and ocular adverse reactions.[1] Bark from the chinchona tree native to the Andes and grown in South America, Indonesia, and Congo containing the quinoline alkaloids quinine and quinidine was the first known source of treatment of malaria.[2] In 1834, quinine was first used to treat systemic lupus erythematosus (SLE).[3] Antimalarial prophylaxis given to soldiers in the Pacific Theater during World War II serendipitously confirmed that this therapeutic class was an effective treatment of arthritis and SLE. Over time, antimalarials have been used to treat patients with numerous rheumatic diseases,

[a] Hospital for Special Surgery, Weill Medical College of Cornell University, New York Presbyterian Hospital, 535 East 70th Street, New York, NY 10021, USA; [b] Department of Ophthalmology, Manhattan Eye, Ear, and Throat Hospital, Zucker School of Medicine at Hofstra/Northwell, Hempstead, NY, USA
* Corresponding author.
E-mail address: ssrheum@gmail.com

Rheum Dis Clin N Am 45 (2019) 359–367
https://doi.org/10.1016/j.rdc.2019.04.008
rheumatic.theclinics.com

including SLE, rheumatoid arthritis, palindromic rheumatism, Sjogren syndrome, and some forms of vasculitis.

Currently, hydroxychloroquine is the predominant antimalarial therapy used in the management of patients with rheumatic diseases. The US Food and Drug Administration has approved this medication for the treatment of SLE, polymorphous light eruption, and rheumatoid arthritis.[4] Hydroxychloroquine has become a critical therapy for patients with SLE and is the drug most widely prescribed for this condition. Importantly, in SLE, it improves survival and has the capacity to prevent disease flares.[5] The rationale for the popularity of hydroxychloroquine is not only that it is effective but also that the risks associated with this medication are very low. Ocular toxicity is an accepted complication of antimalarial therapy. However, monitoring for ocular adverse events is evolving and not universally used according to published recommendations.

Chloroquine was reported to cause retinal toxicity in 1957.[6] This first report by Cambiaggi[6] described retinal findings of a black spot in the macula of both eyes with a small whitish area in the center in a patient with SLE. Discontinuation of chloroquine and initiation of hydroxychloroquine did not result in improvement of the lesion, and the investigators attributed the lesion to active lupus. In retrospect, the published fundoscopic findings were the classic bull's-eye maculopathy due to antimalarial toxicity. In other early reports, 2 patients with retinal damage and constricted visual fields (VFs) in the setting of chloroquine therapy were described.[7] Hydroxychloroquine has since largely replaced chloroquine as the primary antimalarial drug used to treat rheumatologic diseases; however, likewise it is associated with retinal toxicity (**Fig. 1**).

Chloroquine and hydroxychloroquine have affinity for pigmented tissues, particularly in the eye, which is a possible explanation for the ocular toxicity associated with these drugs. With prolonged exposure to hydroxychloroquine or chloroquine, studies in animals demonstrate higher concentrations in the pigmented ocular structures and retina compared with those in other parts of the body.[8,9] Low levels of chloroquine have been detected in plasma and urine, even 5 years after discontinuing the drug.[8]

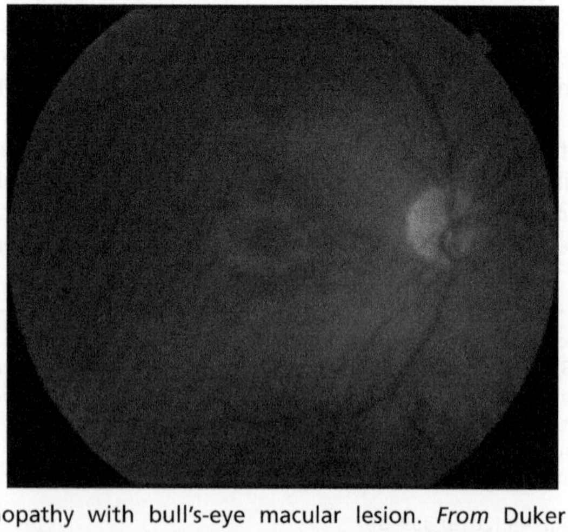

Fig. 1. Bulls retinopathy with bull's-eye macular lesion. *From* Duker JS, Waheed NK, Goldman DR. Hydroxychloroquine Toxicity. In: Handbook of Retinal OCT: Optical Coherence Tomography. Philadelpha, PA: Elsevier; 2014. p. 72–3; with permission.

With current screening technology, hydroxychloroquine toxicity can be detected in advance of obvious retinal damage and visual compromise. Although the ophthalmologist generally assumes primary responsibility of screening for hydroxychloroquine toxicity, it is important for the rheumatologist to have some level of familiarity with which ophthalmologic tests are appropriate and when to use these. Furthermore, it is the rheumatologist's responsibility to assure that proper screening procedures and timing are implemented to assure that retinal toxicity is identified early. Interestingly, a survey study showed that only 5% of rheumatologists and 15% of ophthalmologists were familiar with published screening guidelines.[10] This may be due to the fact that recommendations for monitoring are formulated by ophthalmologists and published in ophthalmology journals rheumatologist screening and self screening by patients using the Amsler grid, a self-administered VF test, has been used in the past but is no longer used because this is an unreliable predictor of toxicity.[11] There is a wide range of methods to screen for ocular toxicity (**Table 1**). Optical coherence tomography (OCT) and VF testing are the current recommended primary screening tests. OCT is a noninvasive imaging test that images the retina in cross-section. The technique uses low-coherence light and is based on low-coherence interferometry. It allows imaging of the entire thickness of the retina with resolution in microns. Its introduction in the 1990s has had a major impact on retinal imaging and has significantly reduced the use of fluorescein angiography and other older testing modalities, such as the Amsler grid, in the diagnosis and management of retinal diseases. Advances in OCT technology have led to increasing resolution of the retina and hence to improved specificity and sensitivity of identifying retinal abnormalities. OCT devices initially were primarily used by retina subspecialists, but, because of their use in both retinal disease and glaucoma, are now commonly used in general ophthalmology practice.

Table 1
Methods to screen for ocular toxicity

Test Name	Description
Visual acuity	Acuity of vision as tested with a Snellen chart; normal visual acuity based on the Snellen chart is 20/20
Color plate testing	Using pseudoisochromic plates with letters or numbers hidden in a maze of dots
Fundus examination	Ophthalmoscopy evaluation of the retina, optic disc, macula, fovea, and posterior pole
Full field ERG and multifocal ERG	Measurement of the electrical activity generated by neural and nonneuronal cells in the retina in response to a light stimulus
Electrooculogram	Measurement of the eye movements through electrodes placed on the skin around the eyes
FAF	A generated image based on the distribution pattern of lipofuscin, which is a fluorescent pigment with a distribution pattern that is disturbed by retinal pathologic condition
Fluorescein angiogram	A retinal image generated by a systemically administered fluorescent dye
OCT	Noninvasive imaging test that uses light waves to take high-resolution cross-sectional tomographic images of the retina
10-2 automated VF testing	VF testing uses fixed points of light, which are shown at different intensity levels, which then correspond to the topographic arrangement of photoreceptors

VF testing was the earliest test used for the screening of antimalarial toxicity. Automated VF testing most commonly tests 30° or 24° of field, but screening for hydroxychloroquine toxicity often focuses on the central 10°, because it is the paracentral foveal region (leading to a paracentral scotoma) that is the most common abnormal early finding. The typical VF examination will be a 10-2 humphrey visual field using a red target, because using red test objects improves the sensitivity of field testing.[12] Asian patients may develop toxicity further from the fovea than do Caucasian patients, and that 10-2 testing would miss early VF changes. Thus, in the Asian population, it is important consider performing standard 30-2 or 24-2 HVF testing.[13]

There are commercially available laboratory tests to measure hydroxychloroquine and its metabolites in whole blood. These tests are infrequently ordered, and, when used, the predominant rationale is either to identify noncompliance or to monitor therapeutic drug levels. In SLE patients, low whole blood hydroxychloroquine concentrations can predict flares and have been associated with active disease.[14] In a study of 300 patients with cutaneous lupus erythematosus, those who failed treatment had significantly lower blood concentrations of hydroxychloroquine than those who achieved complete remission.[15] Because adverse events are very uncommon with this therapy, no studies correlated hydroxychloroquine drug levels with toxicity.

The American Academy of Ophthalmology has published recommendations in 2002, 2011, and 2016 addressing the importance of monitoring for chloroquine and hydroxychloroquine toxicity.[16–18] Interestingly, rheumatologists were not included as collaborators in any of the 3 publications. Systematic literature reviews were not performed; pharmacoeconomic evaluations were not conducted, and patient perspectives were not included. Although several different processes may be used to develop recommendations, such as the Grading of Recommendations Assessment, Development, and Evaluation (GRADE) methodology[19] and Delphi methodology, none was used to develop these recommendations.

In the 2002 recommendations,[16] it was surmised that there was minimal risk of ocular toxicity in patients receiving less than 6.5 mg/kg of hydroxychloroquine or 3 mg/kg of chloroquine for less than 5 years. Therefore, it was recommended that, if a baseline examination was normal, screening be performed over the ensuing 5 years at the frequency of the age-appropriate general ophthalmic recommendations as suggested by the American Academy of Ophthalmology. For example, patients who are between 40 and 64 years old should have an ophthalmologic examination every 4 to 6 years. In addition to the routine examination, the 2002 recommendations suggested that for potential antimalarial toxicity VF and multifocal and full-field electroretinogram (ERG) be performed. This descriptive analysis cited only 12 references, and, although briefly described, none was analyzed critically. These recommendations were based on the opinions of only 5 ophthalmologists who reviewed only descriptive studies.

The 2011 recommendations[17] supported the guideline that a baseline examination be performed, but were more liberal in recommending that screening should then occur after 5 years of use with the caveat that screening should only occur more frequently if other risk factors, such as new visual symptoms, new retinal disease, major weight loss, and liver or kidney disease, were present. Patients who were at increased risk were also identified. These patients were those whose duration of use was more than 5 years, and whose daily dose exceeded 400 mg per day or those who had received more than 1000 mg of hydroxychloroquine. Furthermore, the "elderly," those with prior maculopathy or retinal disease, and those who had kidney or liver dysfunction were identified as being at greater risk of developing retinal toxicity. These investigators recommended that, in addition to 10-2 VF, multifocal

ERG, spectral-domain optical coherence tomography (SD-OCT), or fundus autofluorescence (FAF) be used for screening. Similar to the 2002 guideline, a maximum daily hydroxychloroquine dose of 6.5 mg/kg was recommended. The 2011 recommendations supported the 2002 recommendations but were more definitive in identifying high risks patients and supporting more careful follow up of theses patients. These recommendations were not based on critical data, but rather were presented as the opinion of the authors based on the descriptive studies reviewed.

In a pivotal 2014 publication by Melles and Marmor,[20] the Kaiser Permanente Northern California integrated health organization database was queried using a retrospective case-controlled design. At the time of the study, this organization had electronic medical records on 3.4 million members. Digital ophthalmologic images had been collected since 2009. Inclusion criteria were use of hydroxychloroquine for at least 5 years and having undergone a documented central VF examination or SD-OCT imaging. Exclusion criteria included patients with no evidence of screening, other causes of retinal disease, prior chloroquine use, or those with only fundus examination. Identified were 2361 hydroxychloroquine users, of whom 177 had been diagnosed as having retinal toxicity. The investigators assigned outcomes based on fundoscopic photograph, SD-OCT, and 10-2 pattern deviation and threshold.

The overall prevalence of hydroxychloroquine retinopathy was 7.5%, predominantly in long-term users. This relatively high number was probably due to the fact that modern imaging techniques were able to detect disease much earlier than older diagnostic modalities.[20] Using Kaplan-Meier survival analysis, patients who received a mean daily hydroxychloroquine dose exceeding 5.0 mg/kg had a 10% risk of developing retinal toxicity within 10 years and a 40% risk after 20 years. Patients being treated with hydroxychloroquine doses between 4.0 and 5.0 mg/kg/d had an approximately 2% risk of developing retinal toxicity within 10 years and a 20% risk after 20 years. When patients were treated with hydroxychloroquine at daily doses of less than 5 mg/kg, the risk of developing retinopathy was low at first but then increased with duration of use: from less than 1% during the first 5 years, to less than 2% at 10 years, and to 20% after 20 years. Risk factors for developing retinopathy included higher hydroxychloroquine doses and longer duration of therapy. For those patients receiving hydroxychloroquine doses of more than 5 mg/kg, the development of ocular toxicity was dose dependent. Other major risk factors that were identified included concomitant renal disease, tamoxifen therapy, and prior retinal disease.

There are many recognized risk factors for toxicity. The most important risk factor is daily dose. Studies suggest risk of retinal toxicity is low at dosages of 5 mg/kg (eg, for 70-kg person, 350-mg daily dose) or less. Duration of use is also relevant, with risk increasing with duration of treatment. Annual risk is less than 1% up to 10 years of treatment and increases to around 3% to 4% at 20 years. The presence of renal disease and concomitant use of tamoxifen are identified risks, presumably because of their effect on actual dosage.[21] Other potential factors for increased toxicity include concomitant breast cancer therapy.[22]

Studies have confirmed that retinal damage (and associated vision loss) is less when toxicity is detected early. In a study by Allahdina and colleagues,[23] 22 patients with hydroxychloroquine retinopathy were monitored for 6 to 82 months after drug cessation. Multiple evaluations were performed, and involved eyes were categorized into 4 separate severity stages by qualitative grading OCT. Changes in outcome measures between drug cessation and last follow-up visit were compared between different severity stages. Of the 44 eyes, the distribution noted: stage 1 (subtle changes confined to parafoveal region; n = 14), stage 2 (clear localized changes in parafovea; n = 17), stage 3 (extensive parafoveal changes; n = 7), and stage 4 (foveal involvement, n = 6). Findings revealed that visual acuity measurements across follow-up were stable in stage 1 and stage 2 eyes but decreased significantly in stage 3 and 4 eyes. The investigators concluded that hydroxychloroquine retinal toxicity correlates with retinopathy severity at the time of cessation. After cessation, eyes with only subtle and localized retinopathy were mostly stable, whereas more severely affected eyes continued to progress. Patients with evidence of moderate to severe toxicity have been shown to have progression of retinal damage even after cessation of treatment.[23]

The most recent recommendations published by the American Academy of Ophthalmology in 2016[18] (**Box 1**) were based predominantly on the 2014 publication by Melles and Marmor.[20] The investigators recommended use of 10-2 VF and SD-OCT. A baseline examination was advised as a reference, and annual screening should begin after 5 years. The same risk factors delineated in the prior recommendations were again supported: a daily hydroxychloroquine dose greater than 5 mg/kg, longer duration of use, and renal and hepatic disease (**Table 2**). However, as identified in the Melles and Marmor study, concomitant use of tamoxifen was identified as an independent risk for ocular toxicity. The American College of Rheumatology published a position paper (**Box 2**) that supported the American Academy of Ophthalmology statement.

The recommendation to not use a dose of hydroxychloroquine greater than 5 mg/kg is challenging in that many rheumatologists frequently use a higher dose than recommended. In a study that investigated the use of hydroxychloroquine in the United Kingdom, the Health Improvement Network, an electronic medical record database that represents 6.2% of the UK population, was queried, and 20,933 individuals were identified who initiated hydroxychloroquine between 2007 and 2016. Forty-seven percent of women and 7% of men had excess dosing.[24] In addition, there are inconsistencies in the practices of rheumatologists as they pertain to ophthalmologic screening based on lack of appropriate studies and education. Many rheumatologists recommend at least once yearly ophthalmologic evaluations, and some insist on twice yearly examinations.

The new recommendations were based predominantly on a single albeit robust large retrospective analysis,[20] and there was no input from a rheumatologist. In all probability, none of the investigators had ever prescribed antimalarial therapy and hence were not aware of the needs to adjust therapy in patients with rheumatic diseases. A logistic regression analysis was used to define risk factors, but an analysis of variables, such as individual disease states, ethnicity, and race, was not undertaken. Hydroxychloroquine toxicity was determined based on VF loss or retinal thinning and photoreceptor damage, but not both. Because there currently is no

Box 1
Screening frequency

Baseline screening
- Fundus examination within first year of use
- Add VFs and SD-OCT if maculopathy is present

Annual screening
- Begin after 5 years of use
- Sooner in the presence of major risk factors

From Marmor MF, Kellner U, Lai TY, et al. Revised recommendations on screening for chloroquine and hydroxychloroquine retinopathy. From Ophthalmology. 2011 Feb;118(2):415-22. https://doi.org/10.1016/j.ophtha.2010.11.017.

Table 2
Major risk factors for toxic retinopathy

	Daily Dosage
HCQ	>5.0 mg/kg real weight
CQ	>2.3 mg/kg real weight
Duration of use	>5 years, assuming no other risk factors
Renal disease	Subnormal glomerular filtration rate
Concomitant drugs	Tamoxifen use
Macular disease	May affect screening and susceptibility to HCQ/CQ

Abbreviations: CQ, chloroquine; HCQ, hydroxychloroquine.

From Marmor MF, Kellner U, Lai TY, et al. Revised recommendations on screening for chloroquine and hydroxychloroquine retinopathy. From Ophthalmology. 2011 Feb;118(2):415-22. https://doi.org/10.1016/j.ophtha.2010.11.017.

treatment to reverse the vision loss from hydroxychloroquine retinal toxicity, efforts need to be focused on prevention by appropriate screening. Understanding the impact of daily dosage, duration of therapy, and concomitant risk factors on the development of hydroxychloroquine toxicity has dramatically reduced the incidence of

Box 2
American College of Rheumatology position statement subject: screening for hydroxychloroquine retinopathy

1. Patients beginning therapy should be informed of potential adverse events, including retinal toxicity and that periodic monitoring and early recognition can limit the impact of macular toxicity.
2. All individuals initiating therapy should undergo a complete ophthalmologic evaluation, including the following elements:
   a. Examination of the retina with a dilated examination and VFs by an automated threshold central VF test (Humphrey 10-2).
   b. If available, objective testing, such as multifocal electroretinography, SD-OCT, or FAF testing
   c. If the patient is considered low risk and baseline examination results are normal, no further specialized ophthalmologic testing is needed for 5 years.
3. Some ophthalmologists may elect to screen more often based on the patient's risk factors. Recognized risk factors include the following:
   a. Macular degeneration and retinal dystrophy and cataracts may increase susceptibility to toxicity.
   b. Reduced kidney function.
   c. Tamoxifen use also been identified as risk factors for retinopathy.
   d. Asian patients demonstrate an early pattern of retinal toxicity that is different from patients of European descent.
4. For patients who are considered high risk, annual eye examination is recommended without the 5-year gap.

Presented by: Committee on Rheumatologic Care FOR DISTRIBUTION TO: Members of the American College of Rheumatology Medical Societies Centers for Medicare and Medicaid Services Managed Care Organizations/Third-Party Carriers Arthritis Foundation.

Data from American College of Rheumatology. Screening for Hydroxychloroquine Retinopathy - 08/2016. Available at: https://www.rheumatology.org/Practice-Quality/Administrative-Support/Position-Statements

antimalarial drug eye toxicity. However, for many rheumatologic conditions, the dose of hydroxychloroquine tends to be greater than 5 mg/kg. Further data are required for a more rational approach to screening.

In the future, it will be important to identify other risk factors predisposing to retinal toxicity. New ophthalmic diagnostic tools, such as OCT angiography, can image the retinal microvasculature without the use of an intravenous contrast dye.[25] It is possible that evolving fields, such as pharmacogenetics, will play an important role in defining both potential risk and potential benefit of antimalarial use. The current literature includes only retrospective studies. Hence, a prospective trial comparing different screening paradigms in uniform patient populations could provide further important information. Screening recommendations should be developed by first performing a systematic literature review and then using GRADE methodology and the Delphi method. Existing literature supports the lack of dialogue between rheumatologists and ophthalmologists. Only limited publications have used the perspectives of both specialties.[26] It is critical that both physician groups open a dialogue and develop screening strategies that are based on collaboration.

REFERENCES

1. Rainsford KD, Parke AL, Clifford-Rashotte M, et al. Therapy and pharmacological properties of hydroxychloroquine and chloroquine in treatment of systemic lupus erythematosus, rheumatoid arthritis and related diseases. Inflammopharmacology 2015;23(5):231–69.
2. Schlitzer M. Malaria chemotherapeutics part I: history of antimalarial drug development, currently used therapeutics, and drugs in clinical development. ChemMedChem 2007;2(7):944–86.
3. Dubois EL, Hahn BH, Wallace DJ. Dubois' lupus erythematosus. Philadelphia: Lippincott Williams & Wilkins; 2007.
4. Physicians' desk reference. Montvale (NJ): Thomson PDR; 2005.
5. Ruiz-Irastorza G, Ramos-Casals M, Brito-Zeron P, et al. Clinical efficacy and side effects of antimalarials in systemic lupus erythematosus: a systematic review. Ann Rheum Dis 2010;69(1):20–8.
6. Cambiaggi A. Unusual ocular lesions in a case of systemic lupus erythematosus. AMA Arch Ophthalmol 1957;57(3):451–3.
7. Goldman L, Preston RH. Reactions to chloroquine observed during the treatment of various dermatologic disorders. Am J Trop Med Hyg 1957;6:654.
8. Bernstein H, Zvaifler N, Rubin M, et al. The ocular deposition of chloroquine. Invest Ophthalmol 1963;2(384):384–92.
9. Rosenthal RA, Kolb H, Bergsma D, et al. Chloroquine retinopathy in the rhesus monkey. Invest Ophthalmol Vis Sci 1978;17(12):1158–75.
10. Shulman S, Wollman J, Brikman S, et al. Implementation of recommendations for the screening of hydroxychloroquine retinopathy: poor adherence of rheumatologists and ophthalmologists. Lupus 2017;26(3):277–81.
11. Pluenneke AC, Blomquist PH. Utility of red Amsler grid screening in a rheumatology clinic. J Rheumatol 2004;31(9):1754–5.
12. Percival SP, Behrman J. Ophthalmological safety of chloroquine. Br J Ophthalmol 1969;53(2):101–9.
13. Giocanti-Auregan A, Couturier A, Girmens JF, et al. Variability of chloroquine and hydroxychloroquine retinopathy among various ethnicities. J Fr Ophtalmol 2018; 41(4):363–7.

14. Costedoat-Chalumeau N, Dunogue B, Leroux G, et al. A critical review of the effects of hydroxychloroquine and chloroquine on the eye. Clin Rev Allergy Immunol 2015;49(3):317–26.
15. Frances C, Cosnes A, Duhaut P, et al. Low blood concentration of hydroxychloroquine in patients with refractory cutaneous lupus erythematosus: a French multicenter prospective study. Arch Dermatol 2012;148(4):479–84.
16. Marmor MF, Carr RE, Easterbrook M, et al. Recommendations on screening for chloroquine and hydroxychloroquine retinopathy: a report by the American Academy of Ophthalmology. Ophthalmology 2002;109(7):1377–82.
17. Marmor MF, Kellner U, Lai TY, et al. Revised recommendations on screening for chloroquine and hydroxychloroquine retinopathy. Ophthalmology 2011;118(2): 415–22.
18. Marmor MF, Kellner U, Lai TY, et al. Recommendations on screening for chloroquine and hydroxychloroquine retinopathy (2016 revision). Ophthalmology 2016;123(6):1386–94.
19. Guyatt G, Oxman AD, Akl EA, et al. GRADE guidelines: 1. Introduction-GRADE evidence profiles and summary of findings tables. J Clin Epidemiol 2011;64(4): 383–94.
20. Melles RB, Marmor MF. The risk of toxic retinopathy in patients on long-term hydroxychloroquine therapy. JAMA Ophthalmol 2014;132(12):1453–60.
21. Kim JW, Kim YY, Lee H, et al. Risk of retinal toxicity in longterm users of hydroxychloroquine. J Rheumatol 2017;44(11):1674–9.
22. Sharma AMA, Tucker WR, Cuckras C. Accelerated onset of retinal toxicity from hydroxychloroquine use with concomitant breast cancer therapy. Retin Cases Brief Rep 2018;16:98–102.
23. Allahdina AM, Chen KG, Alvarez JA, et al. Longitudinal changes in eyes with hydroxychloroquine retinal toxicity. Retina 2019;39(3):473–84.
24. Jorge AM, Melles RB, Zhang Y, et al. Hydroxychloroquine prescription trends and predictors for excess dosing per recent ophthalmology guidelines. Arthritis Res Ther 2018;20(1):133.
25. Goker YS, Ucgul Atilgan C, Tekin K, et al. The validity of optical coherence tomography angiography as a screening test for the early detection of retinal changes in patients with hydroxychloroquine therapy. Curr Eye Res 2019;44(3):311–5.
26. Rosenbaum JT, Mount GR, Youssef J, et al. New perspectives in rheumatology: avoiding antimalarial toxicity. Arthritis Rheumatol 2016;68(8):1805–9.

Should Generalized Immunosuppression or Targeted Organ Treatment be the Best Principle for Overall Management of Systemic Lupus Erythematosus?

Nancy Olsen, MD

KEYWORDS

• Biologics • Cutaneous lupus • Immunosuppressives • Lupus nephritis

KEY POINTS

- Systemic immunosuppression offers many therapeutic advantages, and remains the mainstay for many manifestations of SLE, especially for renal involvement.
- Targeted therapies for cellular components of SLE skin lesions have potential for new treatment approaches.
- Targeting organ involvement in an SLE patient is an evolving approach that personalizes care.
- True tissue-specific effects might be achievable by targeting cells that are intrinsic to the involved organ rather than cellular components of immune infiltrates.

INTRODUCTION

Despite major advances in therapeutics for systemic lupus erythematosus (SLE), many gaps remain in the effective management of the protean manifestations of this disease. Mortality in SLE remains unacceptably high and new therapies have been slow to appear. The question of whether modifications in approach to the use of existing or emerging therapeutics might be useful is therefore an important one. Although generalized immunosuppression has been responsible for major therapeutic advances in SLE in the past 50 years, efficacy gaps and adverse consequences still limit applications in many patients. Furthermore, advances in understanding cellular

Division of Rheumatology, Department of Medicine, Penn State M.S. Hershey Medical Center, 500 University Drive, Hershey, PA 17033, USA
E-mail address: nolsen@pennstatehealth.psu.edu

Rheum Dis Clin N Am 45 (2019) 369–377
https://doi.org/10.1016/j.rdc.2019.04.004
rheumatic.theclinics.com

and molecular targets as well as in development of small-molecule and biological therapeutics that can meet these targets present new opportunities.

Targeting therapies can be done in several different ways (**Box 1**). One approach is to target the therapy to the individual patient. The National Institutes of Health precision medicine initiative is designed to find ways to focus therapies using genetic, environmental, and lifestyle information.[1] A second way is to target known pathogenetic mechanisms in a disease. This is a goal of the Accelerating Medicines Partnership, which includes the autoimmune diseases rheumatoid arthritis and SLE as a major area of focus. Current therapeutic targets in SLE include B cells and the type I interferons (IFNs).[2] The present review considers a third targeting strategy, one that is not completely independent of the other two: to target therapy to the involved organ in an individual patient, an approach that is especially relevant to multisystem disorders such as SLE. Organ-targeted therapy might be more useful than generalized immunosuppression in SLE but only with availability of information about organ-specific targets and suitable therapies that match those targets. Furthermore, beneficial effects on the target organ must not be at the expense of off-target damage elsewhere in the treated patient. These are stringent requirements which, if met, could offer new therapeutic breakthroughs with existing or emerging therapies. However, whether this offers advantages over broad immunosuppression is uncertain and is the focus of this review.

Major organs that are involved in SLE include the kidneys, skin, lung, and brain as well as the hematologic and nervous systems. The targeting of therapies to these components of SLE, when possible, would be expected to have the most significant impact on overall disease outcomes. However, each organ-targeted approach has the potential to cause adverse effects elsewhere in this systemic disease. Thus, comparison with the effects of systemic immunosuppression is required to determine whether organ targeting offers potential advantages over a systemic approach. The focus in this review is on 2 organ systems that are most commonly involved in SLE: skin and kidney. Each offers potential local targets while at the same time presenting challenges to make therapeutics act primarily on the locus of disease.

SKIN

Cutaneous manifestations occur in 85% of SLE patients and the types of skin lesions take many forms including discoid, acute, subacute, and other less common variants.[3] Systemic treatment with hydroxychloroquine (HCQ) is highly beneficial for many of the skin lesions of lupus and is considered an essential therapeutic for most SLE patients regardless of organ involvement pattern.[4] Whether HCQ is in fact an immunosuppressant is questionable, but it modulates immune function in a systemic manner through blockade of endosomal toll-like receptors in monocyte/macrophage lineage cells.[5,6] Although HCQ has been demonstrated to have significant benefits in SLE, concerns about retinal toxicity limit its use in some patients. Skin involvement may be also treated topically, which in some ways is an organ-specific form of therapy. In more

Box 1
How therapies might be targeted

To the individual patient, as "personalized medicine"

To the pathogenetic cell, mediator, or pathway

To the organ that is involved

severe cases, the use of systemic and high-dose corticosteroids or immunosuppressives such as azathioprine or methotrexate may be necessary.[7]

However, some SLE patients fail to respond adequately even to these systemic approaches and may require other forms of therapy to prevent systemic consequences, such as infections or permanent scarring. These are cases for which targeting of treatments to the skin manifestations might be of greatest value.[8]

In considering how to effectively administer targeted therapies to the skin, it is helpful to identify the cells, mediators, and pathways that are contributing to the inflammation and damage of cutaneous tissues. A primary target is the B cell, which is a component of the cutaneous inflammatory infiltrate in both cutaneous and systemic forms of lupus. Autoantibodies produced locally by these B cells may engage neighboring targets and have inflammatory and damaging effects.[9] Plasma cells are also seen in skin, consistent with local antibody production.[10] Of note, B cells are seen in active discoid lesions, suggesting a role in this scarring type of lupus lesion.[10] Receptors for B cell stimulating factor are upregulated in discoid skin lesions, and are probably being expressed in these lesions by T cells and macrophages.[11] The B cells and B cell stimulatory pathways can be targeted with available biologics that deplete or alter the functions of B cells, including belimumab and rituximab, both of which have been shown to improve some cutaneous manifestations of lupus.[12,13] These B cell therapeutics, however, have not shown efficacy in discoid lupus erythematosus (DLE), despite the presence of B cells in DLE lesions, suggesting that other cells or pathways may be primarily responsible for the scarring and damage.

Anti-Ro antibodies are a component of the autoantibody response associated with photosensitive skin lesions, and the Ro52 antigen is expressed at high levels in these lesions where it may contribute to the inflammatory process.[14] A relevant investigational agent of interest for cutaneous lupus is RSLV-132, a biologic consisting of human RNase fused to the Fc domain of immunoglobulin (Ig) G1.[15] A small early-phase 1b study was carried out to assess safety and tolerability of RSLV-132 in patients with antibody-bound U1 or Y1 RNA. A total of 32 patients were enrolled in a placebo-controlled, dose-escalation design with a treatment period of 1 month. Although the study was not powered to assess efficacy, an analysis of data from a subgroup of 5 patients who exhibited clinical responses to the treatment revealed decreased levels of the B cell–activating factor BAFF and autoantibodies.[15] The potential use for this biologic in these types of Ro-positive patients is being investigated in ongoing clinical trials.

T cells are present in lupus skin lesions, with an observed predominance of CD4 cells in some specific subtypes such as subacute cutaneous lupus erythematosus, while scarring conditions such as DLE show CD8 predominance.[16] In DLE skin lesions, high levels of CD8 cytotoxic T cells may release intragranular molecules such as TIA-1, with damaging local effects.[9]

Targeting the T cells in lupus skin may be especially useful in the scarring types of lesions. One approach is with lenalidomide, which has been shown to have efficacy in patients with cutaneous lupus refractory to other standard therapies.[16] However, the limited clinical data with lenalidomide suggest that it may at the same time have immunoenhancing effects to activate T lymphocytes systemically, and in at least one case, this triggered systemic manifestations in a patient who was being treated for cutaneous disease. This is an example of how off-target effects might limit efficacy or safety.

T cell responses, especially in the T-helper (Th)1 and Th17 subsets, make use of the JAK/STAT signaling pathway, components of which have been shown to be upregulated in inflammatory skin lesions including cutaneous lupus.[17] The JAK/STAT pathway can be targeted with available agents such as tofacitinib and baricitinib, which are approved by the Food and Drug Administration (FDA) for use in rheumatoid arthritis and alopecia syndromes and for which some preliminary findings suggest may have utility in cutaneous lupus, possibly via a topical approach.[17] Topical use of the calcineurin inhibitor (CNI) tacrolimus is yet another intervention that targets both the cutaneous location and the underlying T cell–mediated inflammatory pathway.

Other drugs may target transcription factors present in both T and B lymphocytes. An example is the cereblon modulator iberdomide, which degrades the transcription factors Ikaros and Aiolos and is useful in the treatment of cutaneous lupus.[18]

Macrophages, identified by their expression of CD68 or CD163, are also present in the skin lesions of SLE, and mediate recruitment of lymphocytes through production of IFN-inducible chemokines including CXCL9, CXCL10, and CXCL11.[16] Blockade of the type I IFN receptor therefore would be anticipated to interfere with chemokines expressed in affected skin lesions. One such investigational agent, anifrolumab, was shown in post hoc analysis of an early-phase (IIb), randomized, double-blind, placebo-controlled clinical trial to improve features of lupus rash in anifrolumab-treated patients.[19] This exploratory analysis suggested the possibility of therapeutic benefit, regardless of whether a patient exhibited elevated expression of the interferon gene signature. Other recently released trial data with anifrolumab unfortunately did not confirm overall efficacy in SLE, but this might be an example of a therapeutic agent that will be useful to treat some, but not all, manifestations of this multisystem disorder.

KIDNEY

When SLE patients develop active lupus nephritis (LN), this clinical manifestation generally drives overall therapeutic decisions. Drugs classically used to treat LN are ones that also generally mediate generalized and systemic immunosuppression, such as cyclophosphamide, azathioprine, and mycophenolate mofetil (MMF).[3] Corticosteroids in high doses also have been used in most of these immunosuppressive regimens, although newer approaches have suggested that a rapid taper of corticosteroid doses improves outcomes.[2,20] There is no question that the use of significant systemic immunosuppression to treat LN has been responsible for the improved survival of lupus patients over the past 3 decades.[21,22] However, these drug regimens also carry significant adverse or off-target effects including cytopenias, infections, and ovarian failure that limit their tolerability and use.

Modifications in protocols using cyclophosphamide have been made to address these concerns. The most notable of these is the lower-dose regimen in the Euro Lupus protocol, which has shown similar efficacy to the high-dose approach with a reduced incidence of the adverse effects of infections and sterility.[23] Several controlled trials have demonstrated that MMF has efficacy similar to cyclophosphamide, and offers fewer adverse effects including the risks of infection and amenorrhea.[24,25] The American College of Rheumatology guidelines for treatment of LN indicate that MMF is preferred to cyclophosphamide as induction therapy for African Americans and Hispanics.[26]

Despite the major advances in treatment of LN that have been made using systemic immunosuppression, the search for new therapies continues. One impetus for this is that a significant number of patients, perhaps up to one-third, still progress to end-stage renal disease.[27] Another is the premise that therapies targeted to specific cells, mediators, or pathways that contribute to LN will be more efficacious. Thus, it is not surprising that many local targets have been proposed and studied in this search for new treatments.

As with skin, a major target within the kidney is the B lymphocyte. A major component of the glomerular injury is mediated by immune-complex deposition and complement fixation, so it is reasonable to look at the B lymphocyte as the source of these antibodies. Although B lymphocyte lineage cells are not typically seen in glomerular infiltrates, memory B cells and fully differentiated plasma cells (PCs) are found in other areas of LN kidneys.[28] The intrarenal PCs in fact make the involved kidney itself a source of antibodies and autoantibodies that contribute to organ damage. This is, in a way, similar to how B cells may function in the skin lesions of SLE, as described in the previous section. Other B cells in the kidney likely contribute to antigen presentation and function as regulatory cells.[29] Of note, the renal-dwelling PCs are long lived and do not cycle actively, making them relatively resistant to the effects of immunosuppressive agents such as cyclophosphamide.

The ability to target the B cell in patients with LN has been facilitated by the availability of biotherapeutics. One of the first of these approaches was to use the anti-CD20 targeting antibody rituximab, which had shown benefits in patients with rheumatoid arthritis. However, rituximab has had only mixed success in LN. The LUNAR (Lupus Nephritis Assessment with Rituximab) trial comprising patients with class III or IV LN did not achieve its primary end point of a complete renal response (normalization of serum creatinine, inactive urinary sediment, and urine protein to creatinine ratio <0.5) at 52 weeks.[30] However, many reports in the literature, including retrospective case series and surveys and observations made in prospective studies of SLE patients, support its value for treatment of LN.[29] Consensus guidelines position rituximab as second-line or third-line therapy after other agents have failed.[26] One limitation of rituximab is that PCs, such as those in the kidneys, do not express CD20 and so would not be targeted for destruction.

Another approach to targeting B cells is with belimumab, a human monoclonal antibody that binds to the B lymphocyte stimulator and shortens the life span of B cells. Belimumab is an FDA-approved therapeutic for patients with SLE. However, as with rituximab, randomized controlled trials did not support the use of belimumab in LN.[29] Overall, it seems that both memory B cells and PCs are more susceptible to effects of generalized immunosuppression with pharmacologic agents such as MMF or cyclophosphamide than with the B lymphocyte–targeted biologics that have been studied in therapeutic trials.[31]

Given that these anti–B cell therapies do not target PCs, other approaches have been proposed to block the pathogenic autoantibodies that are produced. Proteasome inhibitors that have been used in the treatment of multiple myeloma act to interfere with PC function and have shown some efficacy in murine LN models. A small clinical study with the proteasome inhibitor bortezomib in patients with SLE had an unacceptably high number of adverse events requiring discontinuation of the therapy, but other studies with this agent are in progress.[32,33]

Other cellular targets within the kidney include T lymphocytes, which have many relevant functions including production of cytokines, providing helper function for B cells, and as negative regulators in the form of regulatory T cells. In murine lupus models, blockade of T cell coactivation with CTLA4-Ig showed synergistic effects with cyclophosphamide in arresting LN. However, when this approach was tested in a multicenter, randomized controlled trial in patients with SLE, CTLA4-Ig in the form of the biological agent abatacept did not add to the effects of cyclophosphamide, which was a disappointing result.[34]

However, other approaches to T cell blockade for the treatment of LN have shown some promise. One study from China showed benefits of adding the CNI tacrolimus to MMF for induction therapy in LN. More recently a trial using voclosporin, a next-generation CNI with similarities to cyclosporin, showed significant efficacy when used together with MMF for induction of complete renal remission in patients with LN.[20] An excess of mortality in the voclosporin group raised some concerns and remained unexplained but, in the landscape of lupus clinical trials, this one was a rare success and further studies with this drug are in progress. Because the primary target of CNIs is the T lymphocyte, with effects that alter activation and cytokine induction, these data suggest a fundamental role for T cells in LN that might be amenable to other types of therapeutic interventions.

Therapeutic approaches to LN can be developed based on knowledge of pathogenetic pathways, including those that stimulate expression of genes in the type I IFN signature, which is upregulated in peripheral blood of SLE patients and which correlates with features of active disease.[35,36] More relevant to LN is the observation that not only the blood, but also the diseased kidney tissues, may express the type I IFN signature.[37] However, in this study LN renal tissue was found to have great heterogeneity. The LN patients were clearly different from the non-LN controls, but the patients were not very similar to each other. Furthermore, an alternative signature associated with the cytokine tumor necrosis factor (TNF) was found to be more highly expressed during flares than at the time of the initial diagnosis. This raises the possibility that anti-TNF agents might be useful for some LN patients.[38] These observations demonstrate the potential for the immune response to change direction, possibly in response to therapy. Furthermore, these changes may, in part, explain why interventions with agents that block IFN-α or the IFN-α receptor have not been found to have significant benefits in LN. Targeting cytokines in specific organs that are affected by SLE may be difficult to achieve in an individual patient, especially because repeated tissue sampling of organs, such as the kidney, is not clinically feasible.

The kidney also presents the interesting possibility of pursuing a completely different type of organ targeting, focusing on the intrinsic cells of the organ rather than on the cells that make up immune infiltrates. Podocytes and mesangial cells in the kidney produce cytokines, including IL-6 and IL-1β, in response to autoantibodies or immunologic injury, and may mediate local inflammatory effects.[39,40] Delivery of an inhibitor of calmodulin kinase IV, a key factor in the reduced production of IL-2 and in regulatory T cell imbalance in SLE, to podocytes using nanotechnology approaches has been proposed as potential therapeutic approach that takes advantage of these intrinsic cell functions.[39] The potential utility of IL-1β targeting for LN is also suggested by these findings. Given that IL-1β blocking agents are already approved for other human diseases, repurposing these medications to treat LN is an interesting possibility.

SUMMARY

Generalized immunosuppressive therapy for the treatment of SLE has been successful at improving overall outcomes for these patients. Newer biotherapeutics have shifted the therapeutic approach, in part, to targeting cells, mediators, or pathways that are involved in pathogenesis of this disease. The premise of targeting therapy to the involved organ is based on the concept that this would more effectively address the disease pathology while sparing relatively unaffected tissues. Comparing skin and kidney as 2 major organs involved in lupus (**Table 1**), it appears that the tissue-targeting approach is farther advanced for cutaneous than for renal disease.

Reasons for this include the availability of skin for tissue analysis, which allows for identification of specific immune abnormalities to which therapy can be directed. Another advantage of targeting skin is the potential for topical treatments, which likely would have fewer systemic effects. Agents in the CNI class that target T cells are

Table 1
Comparison of skin and kidney as candidates for targeted SLE therapies

Organ or Tissue	Advantages	Disadvantages
Skin	• Topical treatments are possible • Tissue readily available for biopsy and analysis	• Intrinsic skin cell targets are not known
Kidney	• Intrinsic cellular components contributing to pathogenesis, such as podocytes, have been identified	• Tissue is not readily accessible for biopsy and analysis • Surrogate blood markers reflecting intrarenal changes are not available

useful as topicals, and inhibitors of signaling pathways have been proposed.[17] In contrast, renal tissue is relatively difficult to sample, requiring an invasive biopsy that is not without risks. Surrogate markers that reflect the renal pathology are not available. For example, whereas blood from LN patients may show upregulation of the type I IFN signature,[36] the renal tissue shows significant heterogeneity in expression of this pathway and also appears to modulate in response to treatment.[37] Matching a therapeutic agent to the ongoing immune process in the kidney is not yet feasible and, perhaps for that reason, systemic immunosuppressives remain the first-line therapy for LN. However, the kidney offers another intriguing possibility, which is to target intrinsic cells that participate in the immune response, and which may be responsible for early changes in the development of organ damage. If therapeutic agents could be delivered to these cells, it might be possible to minimize or avoid altogether off-target effects or the need for systemic immunosuppression.

REFERENCES

1. Collins FS, Varmus H. A new initiative on precision medicine. N Engl J Med 2015;372(9):793–5.
2. Durcan L, Petri M. Why targeted therapies are necessary for systemic lupus erythematosus. Lupus 2016;25(10):1070–9.
3. Thong B, Olsen NJ. Systemic lupus erythematosus diagnosis and management. Rheumatology (Oxford) 2017;56(suppl_1):i3–13.
4. Ruiz-Irastorza G, Khamashta MA. Hydroxychloroquine: the cornerstone of lupus therapy. Lupus 2008;17(4):271–3.
5. Leadbetter EA, Rifkin IR, Hohlbaum AM, et al. Chromatin-IgG complexes activate B cells by dual engagement of IgM and Toll-like receptors. Nature 2002;416(6881):603–7.
6. Lafyatis R, York M, Marshak-Rothstein A. Antimalarial agents: closing the gate on Toll-like receptors? Arthritis Rheum 2006;54(10):3068–70.
7. Okon LG, Werth VP. Cutaneous lupus erythematosus: diagnosis and treatment. Best Pract Res Clin Rheumatol 2013;27(3):391–404.
8. Deng GM, Tsokos GC. Pathogenesis and targeted treatment of skin injury in SLE. Nat Rev Rheumatol 2015;11(11):663–9.
9. Thorpe RB, Gray A, Kumar KR, et al. Site-specific analysis of inflammatory markers in discoid lupus erythematosus skin. ScientificWorldJournal 2014;2014:925805.
10. O'Brien JC, Hosler GA, Chong BF. Changes in T cell and B cell composition in discoid lupus erythematosus skin at different stages. J Dermatol Sci 2017;85(3):247–9.

11. Chong BF, Tseng LC, Kim A, et al. Differential expression of BAFF and its receptors in discoid lupus erythematosus patients. J Dermatol Sci 2014;73(3):216–24.
12. Hofmann SC, Leandro MJ, Morris SD, et al. Effects of rituximab-based B-cell depletion therapy on skin manifestations of lupus erythematosus—report of 17 cases and review of the literature. Lupus 2013;22(9):932–9.
13. Hui-Yuen JS, Nguyen SC, Askanase AD. Targeted B cell therapies in the treatment of adult and pediatric systemic lupus erythematosus. Lupus 2016;25(10): 1086–96.
14. Ioannides D, Golden BD, Buyon JP, et al. Expression of SS-A/Ro and SS-B/La antigens in skin biopsy specimens of patients with photosensitive forms of lupus erythematosus. Arch Dermatol 2000;136(3):340–6.
15. Burge DJ, Eisenman J, Byrnes-Blake K, et al. Safety, pharmacokinetics, and pharmacodynamics of RSLV-132, an RNase-Fc fusion protein in systemic lupus erythematosus: a randomized, double-blind, placebo-controlled study. Lupus 2017;26(8):825–34.
16. Braunstein I, Goodman NG, Rosenbach M, et al. Lenalidomide therapy in treatment-refractory cutaneous lupus erythematosus: histologic and circulating leukocyte profile and potential risk of a systemic lupus flare. J Am Acad Dermatol 2012;66(4):571–82.
17. Alves de Medeiros AK, Speeckaert R, Desmet E, et al. JAK3 as an emerging target for topical treatment of inflammatory skin diseases. PLoS One 2016; 11(10):e0164080.
18. Schafer PH, Ye Y, Wu L, et al. Cereblon modulator iberdomide induces degradation of the transcription factors Ikaros and Aiolos: immunomodulation in healthy volunteers and relevance to systemic lupus erythematosus. Ann Rheum Dis 2018;77(10):1516–23.
19. Merrill JT, Furie R, Werth VP, et al. Anifrolumab effects on rash and arthritis: impact of the type I interferon gene signature in the phase IIb MUSE study in patients with systemic lupus erythematosus. Lupus Sci Med 2018;5(1):e000284.
20. Rovin BH, Solomons N, Pendergraft WF, et al. A randomized, controlled double-blind study comparing the efficacy and safety of dose-ranging voclosporin with placebo in achieving remission in patients with active lupus nephritis. Kidney Int 2019;95(1):219–31.
21. Bernatsky S, Boivin JF, Joseph L, et al. Mortality in systemic lupus erythematosus. Arthritis Rheum 2006;54(8):2550–7.
22. Zampeli E, Klinman DM, Gershwin ME, et al. A comprehensive evaluation for the treatment of lupus nephritis. J Autoimmun 2017;78:1–10.
23. Houssiau FA, Vasconcelos C, D'Cruz D, et al. The 10-year follow-up data of the Euro-Lupus Nephritis Trial comparing low-dose and high-dose intravenous cyclophosphamide. Ann Rheum Dis 2010;69(1):61–4.
24. Ginzler EM, Dooley MA, Aranow C, et al. Mycophenolate mofetil or intravenous cyclophosphamide for lupus nephritis. N Engl J Med 2005;353(21):2219–28.
25. Dooley MA, Jayne D, Ginzler EM, et al. Mycophenolate versus azathioprine as maintenance therapy for lupus nephritis. N Engl J Med 2011;365(20):1886–95.
26. Hahn BH, McMahon MA, Wilkinson A, et al. American College of Rheumatology guidelines for screening, treatment, and management of lupus nephritis. Arthritis Care Res (Hoboken) 2012;64(6):797–808.
27. Meliambro K, Campbell KN, Chung M. Therapy for proliferative lupus nephritis. Rheum Dis Clin North Am 2018;44(4):545–60.
28. Espeli M, Bökers S, Giannico G, et al. Local renal autoantibody production in lupus nephritis. J Am Soc Nephrol 2011;22(2):296–305.

29. Gregersen JW, Jayne DR. B-cell depletion in the treatment of lupus nephritis. Nat Rev Nephrol 2012;8(9):505–14.
30. Rovin BH, Furie R, Latinis K, et al. Efficacy and safety of rituximab in patients with active proliferative lupus nephritis: the Lupus Nephritis Assessment with Rituximab study. Arthritis Rheum 2012;64(4):1215–26.
31. Schrezenmeier E, Jayne D, Dörner T. Targeting B cells and plasma cells in glomerular diseases: translational perspectives. J Am Soc Nephrol 2018;29(3): 741–58.
32. Alexander T, Sarfert R, Klotsche J, et al. The proteasome inhibitor bortezomib depletes plasma cells and ameliorates clinical manifestations of refractory systemic lupus erythematosus. Ann Rheum Dis 2015;74(7):1474–8.
33. Kohler S, Märschenz S, Grittner U, et al. Bortezomib in antibody-mediated autoimmune diseases (TAVAB): study protocol for a unicentric, non-randomised, non-placebo controlled trial. BMJ Open 2019;9(1):e024523.
34. ACCESS Trial Group. Treatment of lupus nephritis with abatacept: the Abatacept and cyclophosphamide combination efficacy and safety study. Arthritis Rheumatol 2014;66(11):3096–104.
35. Baechler EC, Batliwalla FM, Karypis G, et al. Interferon-inducible gene expression signature in peripheral blood cells of patients with severe lupus. Proc Natl Acad Sci U S A 2003;100(5):2610–5.
36. Feng X, Wu H, Grossman JM, et al. Association of increased interferon-inducible gene expression with disease activity and lupus nephritis in patients with systemic lupus erythematosus. Arthritis Rheum 2006;54(9):2951–62.
37. Mejia-Vilet JM, Parikh SV, Song H, et al. Immune gene expression in kidney biopsies of lupus nephritis patients at diagnosis and at renal flare. Nephrol Dial Transplant 2018. https://doi.org/10.1093/ndt/gfy125.
38. Aringer M, Smolen JS. Therapeutic blockade of TNF in patients with SLE-promising or crazy? Autoimmun Rev 2012;11(5):321–5.
39. Ferretti AP, Bhargava R, Dahan S, et al. Calcium/calmodulin kinase IV controls the function of both T cells and kidney resident cells. Front Immunol 2018;9:2113.
40. Fu R, Guo C, Wang S, et al. Podocyte activation of NLRP3 inflammasomes contributes to the development of proteinuria in lupus nephritis. Arthritis Rheumatol 2017;69(8):1636–46.

Treatment of Antineutrophil Cytoplasmic Antibody-Associated Vasculitis

Is There Still a Role for Cyclophosphamide?

Sebastian E. Sattui, MD[a,*], Robert F. Spiera, MD[b]

KEYWORDS

• ANCA-associated vasculitis • Treatment • Cyclophosphamide • Rituximab
• Remission induction

KEY POINTS

- Use of cyclophosphamide (CYC) , either orally or intravenously, during remission induction phase is effective and generally well tolerated. Intravenous CYC is associated with lower cumulative doses and fewer side effects, with longer-term follow-up but probably higher relapse rates.
- Rituximab is as effective as CYC for remission induction in most cases of microscopic polyangiitis (MPA) and granulomatosis with polyangiitis (GPA) and is more effective for remission induction in relapsing disease. Its role in EGPA is less well established.
- Most of the trials in AAV do not include patients with eosinophilic GPA (EGPA), and generalizability of these trials to EGPA, therefore, is limited.
- CYC still is a reasonable and efficient treatment option for remission induction of generalized severe patients with EGPA with certain manifestations, such as central nervous system involvement and cardiac involvement.
- CYC continues to have a role for remission induction in the most severely ill patients with MPA and GPA, such as those with severe rapid decline in renal function or those with severe alveolar hemorrhage requiring ventilator support.

Disclosures: S.E. Sattui has no disclosures. R.F. Spiera has received research funding from Roche-Genentech, GlaxoSmithKline, Bristol-Myers Squibb, Boehringer Ingelheim, Cytori, Chemocentryx, Corbus, and Formation Biologics and is a consultant to Roche-Genentech, GlaxoSmithKline, CSL Behring, and Sanofi Aventis, Janssen, and Chemocentryx.

[a] Division of Rheumatology, Department of Medicine, Hospital for Special Surgery, 535 East 70th Street, New York, NY 10021, USA; [b] Division of Rheumatology, Department of Medicine, Weill Cornell Medical College, Scleroderma, Vasculitis & Myositis Center, Hospital for Special Surgery, 535 East 70th Street, New York, NY 10021, USA
* Corresponding author.
E-mail address: sattuicortess@hss.edu

Rheum Dis Clin N Am 45 (2019) 379–398
https://doi.org/10.1016/j.rdc.2019.04.006
rheumatic.theclinics.com

INTRODUCTION

Antineutrophil cytoplasmic antibody (ANCA)-associated vasculitis (AAV) represents a group of systemic, necrotizing vasculitides that involve small-sized blood vessels and includes a wide spectrum of organ manifestations. Granulomatosis with polyangiitis (GPA), eosinophilic GPA (EGPA), and microscopic polyangiitis (MPA) are the major clinicopathologic variants described. AAVs are rare, with an estimated worldwide annual incidence ranging from 1.2 to 3.3 cases per 100,000 individuals and a prevalence of 4.6 to 42.1 cases per 100,000 individuals.[1,2] The natural history of AAV used to be progressive and associated with high a mortality, usually in the context of renal or respiratory failure.[3] Currently, the 5-year survival rates for GPA, MPA, and EGPA are 74% to 91%, 45% to 76%, and 60% to 79%, respectively.[4]

Even with the use of glucocorticoids (GCs), morbidity and even mortality in AAV remained high. It was not until the 1970s, when the initial case reports by Fauci and colleagues[5,6] described successful treatment with cyclophosphamide (CYC) and GCs, that prognosis improved.[7] These smaller case series were later followed by large case series that included 85 patients with a follow-up period of 21 years, which showed, through a combination regimen of CYC 2 mg/kg daily and GCs, that complete remission was achieved in 93% of patients.[8] Despite the known toxicities that were later reported by the same investigators and growing literature regarding the management of AAV, CYC changed the landscape of management of these conditions.

Recently, newer agents, such as rituximab (RTX), and newer regimens for remission induction and remission maintenance have been described. The more benign side-effect profiles of these regimens compared with those of CYC have decreased the use of this agent in the management of AAV. This review provides an overview of the literature regarding the management of AAV and highlights the place of CYC in the management of these disorders.

TREATMENT OF ANTINEUTROPHIL CYTOPLASMIC ANTIBODY–ASSOCIATED VASCULITIS

Treatment of AAV should be stratified based on acuity, extent of organ involvement, and severity of disease. The categorization of disease based on severity and extension proposed by the European Vasculitis Study Group (EUVAS) allows guidance in treatment[9] (**Table 1**).

Table 1
European Vasculitis Study Group disease categorization of antineutrophil cytoplasmic antibody–associated vasculitis

Category	Definition
Localized	Upper and/or lower respiratory tract disease without any other systemic or organ system involvement
Early systemic	Any, without organ-threatening or life-threatening disease
Generalized	Renal or other organ-threatening disease, serum creatinine <5.6 mg/dL
Severe	Renal or other vital organ failure, serum creatinine >5.6 mg/dL
Refractory	Progressive disease unresponsive to GCs and CYC

Adapted from Mukhtyar C, Guillevin L, Cid MC, et al. EULAR recommendations for the management of primary small and medium vessel vasculitis. *Annals of the rheumatic diseases.* 2009;68(3):310–317.

In 2015, the European League Against Rheumatism (EULAR) in conjunction with the European Renal Association–European Dialysis and Transplant Association published an update to the 2009 recommendations for the management of AAV.[10] Recommendations for treatment are based on the 2 phases of management, namely a remission induction phase (aimed at achieving clinical remission [CR], which in most recent trials is defined as a Birmingham Vasculitis Activity Score [BVAS] score of 0) and remission maintenance phase. This concept emerged in the wake of the recognition of the substantial toxicities associated with long-term oral CYC use. An important point highlighted by these guidelines is the lack of randomized controlled trials (RCTs) for EGPA, which translate to lower levels of evidence and subsequently lower grades of recommendation, because these are extrapolated from RCTs and studies in GPA and MPA.

CYCLOPHOSPHAMIDE

As a result of initial reports from Fauci and colleagues,[5,8] the use of oral CYC, 1 mg/kg/d to 2 mg/kg/d, combined with GCs became the standard treatment of patients with GPA. CYC was continued for 1 year past CR, whereas GCs were tapered and if possible discontinued after 6 to 9 months. Favorable outcomes were reported, with CR achieved in 75% to 93% in patients with a 5-year mortality rate of 13%.[11] Treatment was associated with a high morbidity due to irreversible features of the disease and/or side effects of treatment. Relapse rates occurred in 30% to 70% of patients, but resuming therapy usually resulted in disease remission.[11,12]

Long-term follow-up studies of these patients showed the significant risks associated with this regimen, including leukopenia, alopecia, infections, infertility, hemorrhagic cystitis, myelodysplasia, and neoplasms.[11] Another study in the same population calculated a 31-fold increased risk for bladder cancer at any age and 51-fold in patients younger than 65 years old compared with the general population.[13]

In an effort to reduce side effects associated with oral CYC, studies comparing use of pulse intravenous (IV) CYC showed comparable rates to that of oral CYC; however, relapse rates were higher.[12,14,15] The Randomised trial of daily oral versus pulse Cyclophosphamide as therapy for ANCA-associated Systemic Vasculitis trial compared pulse IV every 2 weeks to 3 weeks with daily oral CYC for induction of CR in AAV, showing similar rates in achievement of CR (88.1% with IV and 87.7% with orally) as well as the time to remission, relapse rates, cumulative doses of GCs, and deaths. GC regimen was similar in both groups, starting at 1 mg/kg orally and tapered down to 12.5 mg by 3 months and 5 mg by 5 months. Patients in the oral treatment arm had higher CYC cumulative doses as higher rates of leukopenia.[16] Long-term follow-up of this study showed that the risk of relapse was significantly lower in patients in the oral study arm; however, no differences in survival or renal function were noted.[17] No difference in adverse events were noted.

Experience with lower doses of CYC was reported in the CORTicosteroid and cyclophosphamide-based induction therapy for SNV patients AGEd >65 years (CORTAGE) study.[18] This open-label multicenter RCT included elderly patients (over 65 years old) with diagnosis of AAV and polyarteritis nodosa (PAN), who were randomized to either standard management with pulse IV CYC and GCs or a fixed low-dose of pulse IV CYC and GCs (CYC doses were 500 mg/m^2 and 500 mg, respectively). Serious adverse events, the primary outcome of the study, were lower in the low-dose group, and CR rates, deaths, and relapse rates were similar in both groups. Failure of induction with IV CYC and successful achievement of CR with switch to oral CYC were reported in the Wegener's Granulomatosis-Entretien (WEGENT) trial.[19] CR was achieved in 79.2% of patients, but 32 were refractory (GPA 24 and MPA 8). Twenty of these patients were switched to oral therapy and CR was achieved in 15 of them.

Despite its role in severe generalized GPA, experience with effective and safer agents has been reported for the management of early systemic or localized disease. A prospective open-label study of 42 patients without life-threating GPA showed successful achievement of CR with methotrexate (MTX) and GCs in 71% of patients, and reinstitution of treatment was also successful in 75% of patients who experienced a relapse.[20] The patients with diagnosis of glomerulonephritis were followed-up for a median of 76 months, and stable or improved creatinine was noticed in a majority of them.[21] An RCT that included patients with GPA and MPA without early systemic disease and no evidence of end organ damage showed noninferiority of MTX compared with CYC.[22] In patients treated with MTX, delay in CR was noted in patients with more extensive disease and pulmonary involvement as well as higher relapse rate (69.5% and 46.5%, respectively).

All previously discussed studies were focused mostly on patients with GPA and MPA, and EGPA patients were either not included or included in small numbers. One prospective multicenter trial compared the use of different IV CYC protocols, 12 pulses or 6 pulses, in 48 patients with EGPA and at least 1 factor associated with poor outcome.[23] No difference was found between the 2 regimens, with CR achieved in 87.5% of patients. There was no significant difference in total relapses or major relapses between both groups but minor relapses where more frequent in the 6-month treatment group (14 patients vs 6 patients, respectively; $P = .02$). Even though investigators concluded superiority of the 12-month regimen to control severe EGPA, which led to the trial being stopped prematurely, this mostly highlights the importance for remission maintenance therapy.

Remission Maintenance Treatment

Considering concerns for high toxicity with long-term exposure to CYC, agents with a better safety profile were investigated. The first trial to address this issue was the Cyclophosphamide versus Azathioprine for Early Remission Phase of Vasculitis (CYCAZAREM) trial by the EUVAS.[24] This study compared maintenance dosing of azathioprine (AZA), 2 mg/kg/d, to CYC, 1.5 mg/kg/d, in patients with GPA and MPA after achievement of CR with 3 months of oral CYC. After 12 months of therapy, remission maintenance therapy was changed to AZA, 1.5 mg/kg/d, and prednisolone for all patients; 155 (61% GPA and 39% MPA, 94% with renal involvement) patients were included in the induction phase, and 144 patients were randomized to the remission maintenance phase. There were no differences in relapse rates or other outcomes measures including adverse effects, Vasculitis Damage Index (VDI), and deaths.

A more recent single-center open-label trial from Italy randomized 71 patients with AAV (GPA 27, MPA 20, and EGPA 42), after achievement of CR with oral CYC, to either oral CYC (1.5 mg/kg/d) or MTX (goal 0.3 mg/kg/wk, maximum 20 mg/wk) for 12 months of remission maintenance therapy.[25] Patients were followed-up for an additional 12 months. There were no differences in relapse rates, relapse-free survival rates, and adverse events. No differences were noted when GPA, MPA, and EGPA were analyzed separately.

OTHER AGENTS IN THE MANAGEMENT OF ANTINEUTROPHIL CYTOPLASMIC ANTIBODY–ASSOCIATED VASCULITIS

Rituximab

After a successful initial experience reported in open-label trials, 2 large multicenter trials were published in 2010.[26,27] The Rituximab for ANCA-associated Vasculitis (RAVE) trial was a multicenter, double-blind, randomized, noninferiority trial comparing RTX (375 mg/m^2 weekly for 4 wk) with CYC (2 mg/kg/d daily) for remission induction in patients with severe AAV.[28] Both groups were given 1 to 3 methylprednisolone IV pulses of 1 g followed by an oral dose of prednisone 1 mg/kg/d that was tapered during the next 5 months. Inclusion criteria were the following: severe GPA or MPA, newly diagnosed or relapsing disease, age older than 15 years: with active disease defined as a BVAS for Wegener granulomatosis (WG) equal to or above 3 ANCA- proteinase-3 (PR3+) and ANCA- myeloperoxidase (MPO+). Exclusion criteria were patients with limited disease, who were seronegative for ANCA, who had alveolar hemorrhage on mechanical respiratory assistance on enrollment, and with creatinine levels above 4 mg/dL.

The primary outcome was BVAS/WG of 0 and GCs weaning after 6 months was met by 64% of patients in the RTX group and 53% patients in CYC group, meeting the prespecified noninferiority margin. In the subgroup analysis, RTX was superior to CYC for remission induction in patients with relapsing disease. No differences were seen regarding severe flares or adverse events between groups. Remission rates in this trial were low, and this is believed related to the strict GCs tapering regimen in the study design, which mandated tapering corticosteroids off entirely, rather than allowing patients to remain on low-dose corticosteroids. The 18-month extension of RAVE showed no significant differences in relapse, remission, or adverse events rate between both groups. High relapse rates were reported, 77% in the RTX group, and 71% in the control group with a relapse before 18 months, and this was attributed to the early GC weaning. Patients who had a relapse at time of enrollment were analyzed, and RTX was superior at 6 months and 12 months but not at 18 months. RTX patients did not receive treatment with immunosuppressant drugs after induction, showing the importance of remission maintenance therapy.

Ancillary studies from the RAVE trial were focused on relapses. In an analysis on 44 patients with nonsevere relapses between months 1 and 18 treated with steroids, 35% patients achieved remission, but 31 patients (70%) had a second relapse. A shorted timer to second relapse in the RTX group compared with the CYC group (4.7 mo vs 13.7 mo, respectively; $P<.01$).[29] In the analysis of 26 patients with severe relapses, 15 initially assigned to RTX and 11 to CYC, 88% of the patients achieved CR after treatment with open-label RTX.[30] In summary, the RAVE study established that patients presenting with organ-threatening disease, such as those with serum creatinine of greater than 4, dialysis-dependence, or diffuse alveolar hemorrhage requiring mechanical ventilation, have a similar response to RTX compared with CYC for remission induction of newly diagnosed and relapsing patients, with a potential superiority in the latter group.

Rituximab versus Cyclophosphamide in ANCA-associated Renal Vasculitis (RITUXVAS) trial was a European multicenter, randomized, controlled unblinded trial aiming to compare the combination treatment with RTX and CYC versus CYC alone in patients with severe AAV with renal involvement.[31] Inclusion criteria were the following: new diagnosis of AAV (GPA, MPA, or renal-limited vasculitis), ANCA positivity, and renal involvement, as evidenced by necrotizing glomerulonephritis on biopsy or red cell casts or hematuria on urinalysis. The main exclusion criterion was previous use of CYC. Steroid management was similar in both groups, with up to 3 initial pulses of methylprednisolone, 1 g, followed by prednisone, 1 mg/kg/d, with a reduction to 5 mg per day by 6 months. The RTX group received 4 RTX weekly pulses (375 mg/m^2) plus IV CYC (15 mg/kg) with the first and third RTX pulses and no remission maintenance therapy. The control group received IV CYC (15 mg/kg) every 2 weeks for the first 3 doses and every 3 weeks until stable CR, then followed by AZA for remission maintenance therapy. The primary outcome was sustained CR (BVAS/WG 0 for at least 6 months), adverse events, and cancer and death rates. Patients on dialysis were included in this study.

Sustained CR was achieved in 25 of 33 (76%) patients in the RTX/CYC study arm compared with 9 of 11 (82%) in the CYC arm. No differences were noted regarding time to remission, relapse rates at 12 months, and mortality or infection rates. Eight of the 9 patients on dialysis were in the RTX/CYC group; of these, 6 achieved CR and 5 became dialysis independent. In the 2-year follow-up of this trial, there were no differences between both groups regarding the composite outcome of death, end-stage renal disease, and relapse (RTX/CYC 42% vs CYC 36%; $P = 1.00$).[32] No differences were noted when outcomes were analyzed separately.

One single-center retrospective study reported experience with diffuse alveolar hemorrhage in patients with AAV[33]; 73 patients, 47% of them on mechanical ventilation, were reported during a 16-year period. Treatment with CYC or RTX did not show any difference in mortality, length of hospital stay, length of intensive care unit stay, or duration of mechanical ventilation. Treatment with RTX, however, was independently associated with CR at 6 months (odds ratio [OR] 6.45; 95% CI, 1.78–29; $P = .003$).

Two retrospective studies described experiences with the use of RTX for remission induction in EGPA. A multicenter study reported 41 patients with EGPA treated with RTX, either single course or repeated doses, between 2003 and 2013. Patients had refractory, relapsing, or new-onset disease, and clinical presentation was diverse, including patients with cardiac and central nervous system (CNS) involvement; 27 (66%) of these patients had previously used CYC. At 6 months, 83% improved with CR in 34% and partial response in 49%, whereas at 12 months, 49% were in CR and 39% had a partial response.

A single-center retrospective analysis of 28 patients with EGPA, 14 treated with RTX and 14 treated with CYC, showed comparable rates of CR (36% and 29%, respectively). Relapse-free survival was comparable between both groups.

Remission maintenance treatment

The use of RTX for remission maintenance therapy was analyzed in the Maintenance of Remission using Rituximab in Systemic ANCA-associated Vasculitis (MAINRITSAN) study.[34] This RCT was designed to evaluate the effectiveness and safety of RTX-based remission maintenance compared with AZA for remission in AAV. Inclusion criteria for this study were ANCA positivity, histologically confirmed necrotizing small vessel vasculitis, ages between 18 years and 75 years, and newly diagnosed or relapsing GPA, MPA, or renal-limited AAV in complete remission after combined treatment with GCs and IV CYC. AZA was dosed at 2 mg/kg/d for first 12 months, then 1.5 mg kg/d from months 13 to 18, and 1 mg/kg/d from months 19 to 22. RTX was given at a dose of 500 mg, days 0 and 14, and then repeated at months 6, 12, and 18; 58 patients were enrolled in the AZA group and 57 in the RTX group. Major relapses occurred in 17 (29%) patients in the AZA group and 3 (5%) in the RTX group at 28-month follow-up, achieving the primary endpoint. Minor relapses in the RTX group also were noted. No significant differences in adverse events, including infections and malignancy, were noted between treatment groups.

The results of the MAINRITSAN-2 study recently were published.[35] This study included 162 patients, 117 with GPA and 45 with MPA, who were randomized to either a biological parameter tailored RTX regimen of 500 mg or the MAINRITSAN scheduled RTX regimen. Biological parameters studies included $CD19^+$ B lymphocytes and ANCA titers and indication for treatment based on changes in ANCA from previous control (reappearance after being negative, indirect immunofluorescence–determined $\geq$2 dilution-titer increase, and/or at least double enzyme-linked immunosorbent assay PR3 or MPO or $CD19^+$ B-cell count $>0/mm^3$). At month 28, there were no significant differences in the AAV relapse rates between the tailored and fixed-schedule RTX regimens (17.3% vs 9.9%, respectively; $P = .22$), with a significant decrease in the number of RTX infusions in the tailored treatment arm. Flares in setting of negative ANCA titers and/or negative $CD19^{+}$ B-cell population occurred, with 4 (18.2%) patients experiencing 1 or more flares in setting of both ANCA and $CD19^{+}$ B-cell population being negative.

Methotrexate

The Nonrenal Wegener's Granulomatosis Treated Alternatively with Methotrexate (NORAM) study showed that MTX was comparable to CYC for induction of patients with AAV without critical end organ damage and serum creatinine levels less than 150 mmol/L. It was less effective in patients with extensive disease and pulmonary involvement.[22] Previous case series also showed a similar experience for induction, and a positive experience was reported in patients with glomerulonephritis as well.[20,21]

Remission maintenance

Use of MTX, compared with AZA and CYC, for remission maintenance therapy in AAV has been described in 2 different RCTs.[25,36] There were no significant differences among relapse rates between different treatment arms and no difference in adverse events were noted either.

Azathioprine

Remission maintenance

The results reported by the CYCAZAREM trial highlighted the efficacy of AZA for remission maintenance therapy in AAV.[24] Doses recommended in this study range between 1.5 mg/kg/d and 2 mg/kg/d and showed similar recurrence rates to oral CYC.

An open-label RCT compared MTX (0.3 mg/wk, increased to 25 mg/wk) with AZA (2 mg/kg/d) for remission maintenance therapy in AAV patients after induction with IV CYC. Primary endpoint of this study was adverse events requiring treatment discontinuation of the study drug or causing death, and secondary endpoints were severe adverse events and relapse; 63 patients were randomized into each arm, and the primary endpoint was reached in 7 patients in the AZA group compared with 12 patients in the MTX group ($P = .21$). One death was reported in the MTX group. There were no differences in the relapse rates between both groups.

A recent double-blind RCT that included patients with EGPA, MPA, and PAN without poor prognostic factors randomized patients to AZA or placebo to assess benefit of AZA when added to GC monotherapy.[37] The primary endpoint was the combined rate of remission induction failures and minor or major relapses at 24 months; 46 patients were randomized to AZA and 49 to placebo, and at 24 months' remission, induction failures or relapses were reported in 47.8% and 49% of patients, respectively. There was no difference in serious adverse events. In the subgroup analysis of patients with EGPA, no differences were noted in the primary endpoint or incidence of asthma/rhinosinusitis exacerbations between the treatment and placebo group.

Mycophenolate Mofetil

The recently published results of the Mycophenolate Mofetil Versus Cyclophosphamide for Remission Induction of ANCA-Associated Vasculitis (MYCYC) have highlighted the potential use of mycophenolate mofetil (MMF) during the initial phase of treatment.[38] This open-label, randomized, multicenter noninferiority trial randomized 140 ANCA+ patients with newly diagnosed (<6 mo) active GPA or MPA to either MMF (2 g/d with dose increase up to 3 g/d) ot IV CYC. Pediatric patients, 4 in each group, also were included in this study. Oral tapering GC regimen was standard for both groups, and all patients were switched to AZA during remission maintenance phase. Important exclusions from this study included active serious digestive system disease, life-threatening presentations (ie, diffuse alveolar hemorrhage and cerebral or cardiac involvement), patients with rapidly progressive glomerulonephritis and declining renal function, and glomerular filtration rate (GFR) less than 15 mL/min or patients in dialysis. Regarding the primary outcome of remission by 6 months, 67% of patients on MMF achieved remission compared with 61% of patients on CYC achieving noninferiority as per the prespecified margin (absolute risk difference 5.7%; 90% CI, -7.5% to 19%). There were more relapses in the MMF group, and this was accounted for by more relapses in GPA patients. Other secondary endpoints did not differ between groups as well as the report of serious adverse events. Interestingly, 76% of patients in this study received a maximum MMF dose of 2 g, whereas 6% received greater than 2 g and 18% received less than 2 g.

Remission maintenance

The International Mycophenolate Mofetil Protocol to Reduce Outbreaks of Vasculitides (IMPROVE) study was a large open-label RCT developed to test the hypothesis that MMF was more effective than AZA for remission maintenance therapy.[39] This study enrolled 156 patients (76 to MMF and 80 to AZA) in CR after prior induction with CYC and GC. MMF was dosed at 2 g/d. During a median follow-up of 42 months, relapses were more frequent in the MMF group compared with the AZA group (hazard ratio [HR] 1.69; 95% CI, 1.06–2.70; P = .03). Secondary outcomes, such as VDI, serious adverse events, and proteinuria, did not differ between groups. Despite some small evidence of successful remission maintenance treatment with MMF, it is rarely used as maintenance treatment of AAV but may be considered in specific scenarios, such as renal insufficiency precluding MTX use and intolerance of AZA or known thiopurine methyltransferase poor metabolizers.[40]

DISCUSSION

Similar to the impact of CYC in the 1970s to 1980s, the successful use of RTX reported in the RAVE and RITUXVAS trials also represented a major change in the management of AAV. Although RTX has emerged as the favored therapy for remission induction in severe disease, CYC may still have a role in some specific situations that is worth discussing.

Fulminant Generalized Disease

There were important differences between the populations included for both large RTX studies, RAVE and RITUXVAS.[28,31] Patients with alveolar hemorrhage on mechanical respiratory assistance on enrollment and creatinine levels above 4 mg/dL were excluded from RAVE, whereas in the RITUXVAS study, these patients were included in the analysis. In RITUXVAS, however, all patients did receive at least 2 doses of IV CYC, so there were no patients with that degree of severe disease treated with just RTX in either of those trials (they were excluded from RAVE). These differences are clearly evidenced by the 10-point difference in the median BVAS reported in RITUXVAS compared with RAVE. The intervention arm in RITUXVAS (RTX/CYC) showed no difference with regards to sustained CR at 12 months compared with CYC alone. CYC patients then were switched to AZA for remission maintenance therapy. There are some reports of patients with severe presentations (ie, diffuse alveolar hemorrhage with respiratory failure) and successful treatment with RTX compared with CYC but not in RCTs.

Plasmapheresis (PLEX) was usually used in patients with these severe presentations. Besides the MEPEX trial, which showed improvement in renal outcomes at 3 months and 12 months but no difference in survival or adverse events, there were no other RCTs assessing the benefit of PLEX in patients with AAV.[41] The results of the plasma exchange and glucocorticoid dosing in the treatment of anti-neutrophil cytoplasm antibody associated vasculitis (PEXIVAS) trial, a large multinational RCT, recently were presented.[42] The design of this study was to evaluate the effects of PLEX and 2 different regimens of oral GCs in patients with new or relapsing severe AAV. This large trial recruited 704 patients with AAV, 98% with renal involvement and 27% with alveolar hemorrhage; 199 (15%) patients received RTX whereas 595 (85%) received CYC. Even though full results of the study are not yet available, investigators concluded that PLEX did not reduce the risk of end-stage renal disease or death and that reduced GCs did not substantially increase the risk of either.

Specific Organ Involvement

Central nervous system

CNS manifestations (pituitary involvement, meningeal involvement, and cerebral vasculitis) are rare and usually underrepresented in trials.[43] These presentations are associated with significant morbidity and permanent damage. Treatment is guided mostly by experiences reported in case reports and small case series.[44,45] There is experience with both CYC and RTX for remission induction, but, due to CYC being more widely used, there is more information about outcomes with that therapy.[44] One retrospective case series of patients with GPA (5 with white matter ischemic lesions, 2 with hypertrophic pachymeningitis, 1 with orbital pseudotumor, and 1 with mastoiditis and bilateral facial nerve palsy) reported CR in 6 of 9 (66.7%) and 1 death. All but 1 patient were treated with CYC. Relapse rates were 1.812 per 100 person-months. Two of the 8 patients had residual neurologic deficit.

A retrospective study of 26 patients with EGPA and CNS involvement reported experience with treatment and analyzed 62 cases reported in the literature.[46] CYC was used in 63% of cases. Among 81 patients with available data, complete response was observed in 43%, partial response in 43%, and no response in 14%; 56 of 81 patients (57%) had persistent neurologic sequelae.

Otolaryngologic

CYC is not used routinely in patients with ear, nose, and throat (ENT) involvement in GPA. Most of the data for this form of limited disease focus on the use of MTX, AZA, and trimethoprim-sulfamethoxazole (TMP-SMX). Reports of CYC for refractory cases of ENT manifestations, however, exist. A retrospective cohort study of 99 GPA patients with ENT manifestations compared patients who had received RTX (51 patients with at least 1 dose) to patients (48 patients) treated with other agents (MTX, AZA, CYC, and TMP-SMX).[47] Remission of ENT disease was seen in 92.4% of patients treated with RTX compared with 53.7% of treated with other agents. Patients receiving RTX were 11 time (OR 11.0; 95% CI, 5.5–22.0) more likely to achieve remission in the ENT domain during the follow-up time.

With regard to treatment in the remission maintenance phase of AAV, CYC's role has been supplanted by other agents, such as MTX and AZA (**Table 2**). Also, the MAINRITSAN and MAINRITSAN-2 studies supported a role for RTX in remission maintenance. This concept also is being evaluated in the ongoing Rituximab Versus Azathioprine as Therapy ror Maintenance of Remission for Antineutrophil Cytoplasm Antibody-Associated Vasculitis (RITAZAREM) study.[48]

Eosinophilic Granulomatosis with Polyangiitis

Treatment of EGPA is limited by the scant data available in terms of prospective double-blinded trials. Most of the recommendations for its management are inferred

Table 2
Randomized controlled trials in remission induction and remission maintenance in antineutrophil cytoplasmic antibody–associated vasculitis

Trial, Author, and Year	Rationale/Question Behind Study	Design and Subjects	Inclusion and Exclusion Criteria	Intervention	Primary Outcomes	Secondary Outcomes
Remission induction						
MYCYC, EUVAS, Jones et al,[38] 2019	MMF for remission induction in AAV	Multicenter, open label n = 140 6-mo follow-up Noninferiority	IC: new diagnosis GPA or MPA (<6 mo), ANCA+ or positive biopsy, active disease (1 major or 3 minor BVAS criteria) EC: serious GI disease, life-threating presentations (ie, DAH), rapidly progressive glomerulonephritis, CrCl <15 mL/min or dialysis	MMF (2 g/d with dose increase up to 3 g/d) vs IV CYC (15 mg/kg, every 2–3 wk). GC per protocol Maintenance with AZA	Remission 6 mo: 67% MMF vs 61% CYC, achieving noninferiority	More relapses in MMF group No difference between SAE or other secondary endpoints, including VDI and cumulative GC dosing
CORTAGE, FVSG, Pagnoux et al,[18] 2015	Safety of low-dose IV CYC vs standard dosing	Multicenter, open label n = 104, ≥65 y 36-mo follow-up	IC: new diagnosis PAN, EGPA, GPA or MPA, ACR, and/or CHCC criteria, ≥65 y EC: no prior CYC or other immunosuppressant, GCs <1 mo prior	IV CYC 500 mg every 2–3 wk for 6 doses + 9 mo of GCs vs IV CYC 500 mg/m^2 + 26 mo of GCs Maintenance with AZA, MTX or MMF	Occurrence of SAE, including deaths: no differences (60% vs 78%; *P* = .04)	No difference in remission rates More releases noted in low-dose CYC group (44% vs 29%; *P* = .15)

RAVE, Stone et al,[28] 2010	RTX for remission induction in AAV	Multicenter, double-blind n = 197 Noninferiority 6-mo follow-up	IC: new diagnosis or relapsing severe GPA or MPA, >15 y, BVAS/WG $\geq$3, ANCA+ EC: limited disease, ANCA−, alveolar hemorrhage on mechanical respiratory assistance, SCr creatinine >4 mg/dL	RTX 375 mg/m^2/wk × 4 vs CYC 2 mg/kg/d GC per protocol	Remission 6 mo with GC taper: RTX was noninferior (64% vs 53%; *P*<.01)	No differences in steroid dose at 12 mo, relapse rate, SF-36 score RTX was superior in inducing remission in relapsing disease (67% vs 42%; *P* = .01)
RITUXVAS, EUVAS, Jones et al,[31] 2010	RTX-CYC regimen for remission induction in AAV	Multicenter, open label n = 44 Randomization RTX:CYC 3:1 12-mo follow-up	IC: new diagnosis GPA or MPA, ANCA+, renal involvement (hematuria or biopsy) EC: previous use of CYC	RTX 375 mg/m^2/wk × 4 plus IV CYC (15 mg/kg) with first and third RTX pulses, no remission maintenance therapy, vs IV CYC (15 mg/kg) every 2 wk for the first 3 doses and every 3 wk, followed by AZA GC per protocol	Remission 12 mo: no differences (RTX 76% vs CYC 82%; *P* = .68)	No differences in steroid dose, relapses, quality of life (SF-36). No difference in SAE Two-year follow-up did not show any difference in composite of death, ESRD and relapse.

(*continued on next page*)

Table 2
(continued)

Trial, Author, and Year	Rationale/Question Behind Study	Design and Subjects	Inclusion and Exclusion Criteria	Intervention	Primary Outcomes	Secondary Outcomes
CYCLOPS, EUVAS, de Groot et al,[16] 2009	IV CYC vs oral CYC for remission induction in AAV	Multicenter, open label n = 149 18-mo follow-up	IC: GPA, MPA, or RLV; renal involvement (SCr >150 mmol/L and ≤500 mmol/L, biopsy with necrotizing glomerulonephritis, red blood cell casts or hematuria, proteinuria >1 g/d); ANCA+ EC: coexisting autoimmune condition, SCr >500 mmol/L, previous cancer, ages <18 and >75.	IV CYC (15 mg/kg) every 2 wk × 3, followed by pulses at 3 wk-intervals vs oral CYC 2 mg/kg/d Maintenance with AZA	Time to remission: no difference (HR 1.098; 95% CI, 0.78–1.55; *P* = .59)	Patients on CR at 9 mo: 88.1% vs 87.7% No difference in survival, AEs Trend toward higher relapse rates in IV CYC (17% IV vs 8% PO) More leukopenia in oral CYC, no difference in infections
FVSG/EUVAS, Cohen et al,[23] 2007	Determine shortest immunosuppressant regimen with IV CYC for EGPA	Multicenter, open label n = 48 8 y	IC: recent diagnosis of EGPA and at least 1 of the following: SCr >140 mmol/L, proteinuria >1 gm/d, CNS, GI, and cardiac involvement EC: relapsing or previously treated EGPA, age <18 y, history of cancer of human immunodeficiency virus	6 vs 12 IV CYC pulses (dose 0.6 gm/m^2, every 2 wk for 1 mo and then every 4 wk)	Remission rates: no difference 91.3% vs 84%.	Relapses were more frequent in 6-pulse group (73.8% vs 61.9%; *P* = .07). Minor relapses more frequent in 6-pulse group. No differences in side effects

NOMAD, EUVAS, De Groot et al,[22] 2005	MTX use for remission induction of in early AAV	Multicenter, open label Noninferiority n = 100 18-mo follow-up	IC: GPA or MPA with involvement of 1 or more organ and constitutional symptoms, ANCA+, or nonrenal biopsy showing neutrophil infiltrate and/or SVNV EC: organ or life-threatening manifestations, SCr >150 mmol/L, red cell casts or proteinuria >1gm/d, skin vasculitis only, coexisting autoimmune condition, ages <18 and >75.	MTX 15 mg/wk increasing to max 20–25 mg/wk vs CYC 2 mg/kg/d (reduced to 1.5 mg/kg/d at remission)	Remission at 6 mo: 89.8% in MTX vs 93.5% in CYC, proving noninferiority ($P = .04$)	Time to remission: similar in both groups but delayed in MTX group for patients more extensive disease or pulmonary involvement. Relapse rates higher in MTX (69.5% vs 45.5%)
Remission maintenance						
MAINRITSAN-2, FVSG, Charles et al,[35] 2018	Remission maintenance with RTX dosing based on criteria of immunologic recurrence	Multicenter, open label n = 162 28-mo follow-up	IC: new diagnosis GPA or MPA, >18 y, in remission (BVAS 0) after induction (with CYC, RTX, MTX) EC: another vasculitis, induction with nonrecommended agent, history of cancer in 5 y prior	RTX 500 mg at baseline and during recurrence of immunologic ($CD19^+$ B cells or ANCA status) vs RTX 500 mg at days 0 and 14 followed by 6 mo, 12 mo, and 18 mo	Relapses at mo 28: no differences between tailored infusion and fixed-schedule (17.3% vs 9.9%; $P = .22$).	No differences in relapse-free survival rates, VDI and adverse events Tailored infusion vs fixed-schedule received 248 vs 381 infusions, respectively

(continued on next page)

Table 2
(continued)

Trial, Author, and Year	Rationale/Question Behind Study	Design and Subjects	Inclusion and Exclusion Criteria	Intervention	Primary Outcomes	Secondary Outcomes
Maritati et al,[25] 2017	MTX for remission maintenance in AAV	Single center, open label n = 71 24-mo follow-up Early termination due to slow enrolment	IC: clinically active GPA, EGPA (with FFS $\geq$1) or MPA, ages 18–80 EC: other systemic autoimmune disease, eGFR <10 mL/min/1.73 m^2	PO MTX dose 0.3 mg/kg/wk (maximum 20 mg/wk) vs CYC 1.5 mg/kg/d Induction with 3 CS pulses and oral GCs and oral CYC	Relapse rate: no difference in rate by 12 mo (8% in MTX vs 9% in CYC; *P* = 1.00)	No differences in relapse rate at 6 mo and 12 mo, no difference in adverse events
CHUSPAN2, FVSG, Puechal et al,[37] 2017	Addition of AZA to GCs to achieve higher sustained remission of nonsevere EGPA, MPA, and PAN	Multicenter, double-blind n = 101 24-mo follow-up	IC: EGPA, MPA, or PAN with no FFS poor prognosis items, no DAH, enrolled within 3 wk after starting GCs (EGPA up to 1 mo) EC: other vasculitis or taking another immunosuppressant	AZA 2 mg/kg/d vs placebo after initial tapering off steroids during initial 12 mo	Combined rate of remission induction failures and minor or major relapses at 24 mo: 47.8% in AZA vs 49% in placebo (*P* = .86)	No differences in initial remission rate, total relapse rate and GC use
REMAIN, EUVAS, Karras et al,[51] 2017	Determine shortest duration of remission maintenance with AZA/GCs for relapse prevention	Multicenter, open label n = 121 24-mo follow-up	IC: GPA, MPA, or RLV, renal or other organ damage, ANCA+ or ANCA− with positive biopsy, remission induction with CYC for 3 mo, stable remission. EC: previous life-threatening relapse, ESRD	Continuation group: AZA/GC for 48 mo vs withdrawal group: AZA/GC for 24 mo	Relapse risk: 63% in withdrawal vs 22% continuation group (*P*<.0001; OR 5.96; 95% CI, 2.58–13.77)	Major relapses were more frequent in withdrawal group (35.3% vs 13.5%). No difference in eGFR by time of last follow-up. No significant difference in AE between both groups

MAINRITSAN, FVSG, Guillevin et al,[52] 2014	Low-dose RTX for maintenance in AAV	Multicenter, open label n = 115 28-mo follow-up	IC: new diagnosis GPA or MPA, >18 y, in remission (BVAS 0) after induction with CYC, ANCA+ or positive biopsy EC: previously received RTX or another biologic therapy	RTX 500 mg at days 0 and 14 followed by 6 mo, 12 mo, and 18 mo vs AZA (2 mg/kg/d for 12 mo, 1.5 mg/kg/d for 6 mo, 4 mg/kg/d for 4 mo) Remission induction with GCs and IV CYC pulses	Major relapses at 28 mo: reduced rate of relapse with RTX (38% vs 55%; *P* = .03).	No differences in SAEs, VDI, eGFR, proteinuria
IMPROVE, EUVAS, Hiemstra et al,[39] 2010	MMF for remission maintenance and relapse prevention in AAV	Multicenter, open label 156 subjects 48 mo–51 mo follow-up	IC: new diagnosis GPA or MPA fulfilling CHCC, age 18–75 y, ANCA+ EC: previous exposure to cytotoxic drugs, coexistence of other autoimmune disease	AZA 2 mg/kg/d (reduced to 1.5 mg/kg/d at 12 mo, 1 mg/kg/d at 18 mo, withdrawn at 42 mo) vs MMF 2 g/d (reduced to 1.5 g/d at 12 mo, 1 g/d at 18 mo and withdrawn at 42 mo) Induction regimen with CYC and GC, and GC tapering regimen	Relapse-free survival: reduced rate with AZA (38% vs 55%; *P* = .03)	No differences in SAEs, VDI, eGFR and proteinuria

(*continued on next page*)

Table 2
(*continued*)

Trial, Author, and Year	Rationale/Question Behind Study	Design and Subjects	Inclusion and Exclusion Criteria	Intervention	Primary Outcomes	Secondary Outcomes
WEGENT, FVSG, Pagnoux et al,[36] 2008	Safety and efficacy of MTX and AZA for remission maintenance in AAV	Multicenter, open label 126 subjects 29-mo follow-up	IC: new diagnosis GPA (patients with renal involvement, involvement of at least 2 organs or 1 organ and constitutional symptoms) or MPA ($\geq$1 item of FFS), positive pathology and ANCA+ EC: GCs for more than 1 moth prior to induction with CYC, coexistence of other autoimmune disease	AZA 2 mg/kg/d vs MTX 0.3 mg/kg/wk (goal 25 mg/wk) Remission induction with IV CYC and GC Maintenance therapies were withdrawn after 12-mo follow-up	Incidence of AE causing death of leading to discontinuation of drug: no difference 11% AZA vs 19% MTX (P = .21)	No differences in relapse rate (36% AZA vs 33% MTX; P = .71) or relapse-free survival at 24 mo (71.8% AZA vs 74.5 MTX) 73% of patients experienced a relapse after discontinuation of study drug
CYCAZAREM, EUVAS, Jayne et al,[24] 2003	Relapse prevention with AZA in AAV and reduction of CYC exposure	Multicenter, open label 144 subjects 18-mo follow-up	IC: GPA, MPA, or RLV; renal involvement or another end organ damage, ANCA+ (ANCA− if positive biopsy) EC: use of cytotoxic drug within previous year, coexistence of other autoimmune disease, SCr >5.7 mg/dL, age <18 and >75	AZA 2 mg/kg/d vs oral CYC 1.5 mg/kg/d Both groups switched to AZA 1.5 mg/kg/d at 12 mo Remission induction with oral CYC and GC	Relapse, either major or minor: no difference 16% AZA vs 14% CYC (P = .65)	No difference in SAE, recovery of renal function, BVAS, VDI, or SF-36 between groups

Abbreviations: ACR, American College of Rheumatology; AE, adverse events; CHCC, Chapel Hill Consensus Conference; CHUSPAN2, evaluation of a new treatment strategy for patients with microscopic polyangiitis, polyarteritis nodosa [PAN] or eosinophilic granulomatosis with polyangiitis [Churg-Strauss Syndrome] without poor prognosis factors; CrCl, creatinine clearance; DAH, diffuse alveolar hemorrhage; eGFR, estimated GFR; EC, exclusion criteria; ESRD, end-stage renal disease; FFS, five-factor score; FVSG, French Vasculitis Study Group; GI, gastrointestinal; IC, inclusion criteria; RLV, renal limited vasculitis; SAE, serious adverse events; SCr, serum creatinine; SF-36, 36-item short form health survey; SVNV, small vessel necrotizing vasculitis.

from larger trials that included only GPA and MPA patients or from descriptive or retrospective analyses. As discussed previously, there is only 1 trial that enrolled patients with EGPA and poor prognosis factors. This study assessed a 12-month to a 6-month regimen of IV CYC (ie, 12 vs 6 IV pulses), with results favoring treatment with a 12-month regimen based on the lower relapse rate in this treatment arm.[23]

In 2015, The EGPA Consensus Task Force recommendations for evaluation and management still favored another immunosuppressant besides GCs for life and/or organ-threatening disease manifestations, and CYC was the preferred agent.[49] This recommendation was graded as moderate quality of evidence. Use of RTX also was recommended but in selected ANCA+ patients with renal involvement or refractory disease. This recommendation also supported considering RTX in patients where the use of CYC was undesirable (ie, fertility concerns or concern for high cumulative CYC dose). Cardiac involvement, which usually occurs in ANCA- patients with severe eosinophilia, is a complication associated with high morbidity and mortality. Most of the reported experience in the successful treatment of this complication is with CYC; therefore, CYC generally remains the favored treatment of patients with this disease manifestation.[50]

SUMMARY

Over the past decade, understanding of AAV has resulted in a dramatic improvement in the treatment and outcomes. The introduction of oral CYC into the management of AAV marked the first step into improving the treatment of AAV and long-term outcomes of a disease that previously carried a survival of only a few years. Treatment with oral CYC was limited due to the significant side effects and morbidity associated with higher cumulative doses, and IV pulses CYC became more widely used due to concern for lower total doses. New immunosuppressive agents, such as AZA and MTX, showed efficacy during the remission maintenance phase, and the landmark RAVE and RITUXVAS trials highlighted the use of RTX in for remission induction in AAV.

Due to the availability of effective and safer agents, CYC has no role in treatment during the remission maintenance phase. Despite encouraging results of trials using RTX, CYC still has a role in the management of patients with generalized severe disease, CNS involvement, and severe presentations of EGPA, including cardiac involvement. Despite the concerns with side effects, the use of CYC restricted to the remission induction phase has shown an acceptable safety profile, as seen in all large RCTs. More widespread use of RTX may still be limited by the very high direct financial costs of that treatment strategy. In these scenarios, and if accompanied by close monitoring of side effects and prevention of other side effects, such as infertility, CYC continues to be an effective and safe option in the management of AAV.

REFERENCES

1. Berti A, Cornec D, Crowson CS, et al. The epidemiology of antineutrophil cytoplasmic autoantibody-associated vasculitis in olmsted county, minnesota: a twenty-year us population-based study. Arthritis Rheumatol 2017;69(12): 2338–50.
2. Watts RA, Mahr A, Mohammad AJ, et al. Classification, epidemiology and clinical subgrouping of antineutrophil cytoplasmic antibody (ANCA)-associated vasculitis. Nephrol Dial Transplant 2015;30(Suppl 1):i14–22.
3. Walton EW. Giant-cell granuloma of the respiratory tract (Wegener's granulomatosis). Br Med J 1958;2(5091):265–70.

4. Mukhtyar C, Flossmann O, Hellmich B, et al. Outcomes from studies of antineutrophil cytoplasm antibody associated vasculitis: a systematic review by the European League Against Rheumatism systemic vasculitis task force. Ann Rheum Dis 2008;67(7):1004–10.
5. Fauci AS, Wolff SM. Wegener's granulomatosis: studies in eighteen patients and a review of the literature. Medicine 1973;52(6):535–61.
6. Fauci AS, Wolff SM, Johnson JS. Effect of cyclophosphamide upon the immune response in Wegener's granulomatosis. N Engl J Med 1971;285(27):1493–6.
7. Novack SN, Pearson CM. Cyclophosphamide therapy in Wegener's granulomatosis. N Engl J Med 1971;284(17):938–42.
8. Fauci AS, Haynes BF, Katz P, et al. Wegener's granulomatosis: prospective clinical and therapeutic experience with 85 patients for 21 years. Ann Intern Med 1983;98(1):76–85.
9. Mukhtyar C, Guillevin L, Cid MC, et al. EULAR recommendations for the management of primary small and medium vessel vasculitis. Ann Rheum Dis 2009;68(3):310–7.
10. Yates M, Watts RA, Bajema IM, et al. EULAR/ERA-EDTA recommendations for the management of ANCA-associated vasculitis. Ann Rheum Dis 2016;75(9):1583–94.
11. Hoffman GS, Kerr GS, Leavitt RY, et al. Wegener granulomatosis: an analysis of 158 patients. Ann Intern Med 1992;116(6):488–98.
12. Guillevin L, Cordier JF, Lhote F, et al. A prospective, multicenter, randomized trial comparing steroids and pulse cyclophosphamide versus steroids and oral cyclophosphamide in the treatment of generalized Wegener's granulomatosis. Arthritis Rheum 1997;40(12):2187–98.
13. Talar-Williams C, Hijazi YM, Walther MM, et al. Cyclophosphamide-induced cystitis and bladder cancer in patients with Wegener granulomatosis. Ann Intern Med 1996;124(5):477–84.
14. Reinhold-Keller E, Kekow J, Schnabel A, et al. Effectiveness of cyclophosphamide pulse treatment in Wegener's granulomatosis. Adv Exp Med Biol 1993;336:483–6.
15. Hoffman GS, Leavitt RY, Fleisher TA, et al. Treatment of Wegener's granulomatosis with intermittent high-dose intravenous cyclophosphamide. Am J Med 1990;89(4):403–10.
16. de Groot K, Harper L, Jayne DR, et al. Pulse versus daily oral cyclophosphamide for induction of remission in antineutrophil cytoplasmic antibody-associated vasculitis: a randomized trial. Ann Intern Med 2009;150(10):670–80.
17. Harper L, Morgan MD, Walsh M, et al. Pulse versus daily oral cyclophosphamide for induction of remission in ANCA-associated vasculitis: long-term follow-up. Ann Rheum Dis 2012;71(6):955–60.
18. Pagnoux C, Quemeneur T, Ninet J, et al. Treatment of systemic necrotizing vasculitides in patients aged sixty-five years or older: results of a multicenter, open-label, randomized controlled trial of corticosteroid and cyclophosphamide-based induction therapy. Arthritis Rheumatol 2015;67(4):1117–27.
19. Seror R, Pagnoux C, Ruivard M, et al. Treatment strategies and outcome of induction-refractory Wegener's granulomatosis or microscopic polyangiitis: analysis of 32 patients with first-line induction-refractory disease in the WEGENT trial. Ann Rheum Dis 2010;69(12):2125–30.
20. Sneller MC, Hoffman GS, Talar-Williams C, et al. An analysis of forty-two Wegener's granulomatosis patients treated with methotrexate and prednisone. Arthritis Rheum 1995;38(5):608–13.

21. Langford CA, Talar-Williams C, Sneller MC. Use of methotrexate and glucocorticoids in the treatment of Wegener's granulomatosis. Long-term renal outcome in patients with glomerulonephritis. Arthritis Rheum 2000;43(8):1836–40.
22. De Groot K, Rasmussen N, Bacon PA, et al. Randomized trial of cyclophosphamide versus methotrexate for induction of remission in early systemic antineutrophil cytoplasmic antibody-associated vasculitis. Arthritis Rheum 2005;52(8): 2461–9.
23. Cohen P, Pagnoux C, Mahr A, et al. Churg-Strauss syndrome with poor-prognosis factors: a prospective multicenter trial comparing glucocorticoids and six or twelve cyclophosphamide pulses in forty-eight patients. Arthritis Rheum 2007; 57(4):686–93.
24. Jayne D, Rasmussen N, Andrassy K, et al. A randomized trial of maintenance therapy for vasculitis associated with antineutrophil cytoplasmic autoantibodies. N Engl J Med 2003;349(1):36–44.
25. Maritati F, Alberici F, Oliva E, et al. Methotrexate versus cyclophosphamide for remission maintenance in ANCA-associated vasculitis: a randomised trial. PLoS One 2017;12(10):e0185880.
26. Keogh KA, Ytterberg SR, Fervenza FC, et al. Rituximab for refractory Wegener's granulomatosis: report of a prospective, open-label pilot trial. Am J Respir Crit Care Med 2006;173(2):180–7.
27. Keogh KA, Wylam ME, Stone JH, et al. Induction of remission by B lymphocyte depletion in eleven patients with refractory antineutrophil cytoplasmic antibody-associated vasculitis. Arthritis Rheum 2005;52(1):262–8.
28. Stone JH, Merkel PA, Spiera R, et al. Rituximab versus cyclophosphamide for ANCA-associated vasculitis. N Engl J Med 2010;363(3):221–32.
29. Miloslavsky EM, Specks U, Merkel PA, et al. Outcomes of nonsevere relapses in antineutrophil cytoplasmic antibody-associated vasculitis treated with glucocorticoids. Arthritis Rheumatol 2015;67(6):1629–36.
30. Miloslavsky EM, Specks U, Merkel PA, et al. Rituximab for the treatment of relapses in antineutrophil cytoplasmic antibody-associated vasculitis. Arthritis Rheumatol 2014;66(11):3151–9.
31. Jones RB, Tervaert JW, Hauser T, et al. Rituximab versus cyclophosphamide in ANCA-associated renal vasculitis. N Engl J Med 2010;363(3):211–20.
32. Jones RB, Furuta S, Tervaert JW, et al. Rituximab versus cyclophosphamide in ANCA-associated renal vasculitis: 2-year results of a randomised trial. Ann Rheum Dis 2015;74(6):1178–82.
33. Cartin-Ceba R, Diaz-Caballero L, Al-Qadi MO, et al. Diffuse alveolar hemorrhage secondary to antineutrophil cytoplasmic antibody-associated vasculitis: predictors of respiratory failure and clinical outcomes. Arthritis Rheumatol 2016;68(6): 1467–76.
34. Pagnoux C, Guillevin L. Rituximab or azathioprine maintenance in ANCA-associated vasculitis. N Engl J Med 2015;372(4):386–7.
35. Charles P, Terrier B, Perrodeau E, et al. Comparison of individually tailored versus fixed-schedule rituximab regimen to maintain ANCA-associated vasculitis remission: results of a multicentre, randomised controlled, phase III trial (MAINRITSAN2). Ann Rheum Dis 2018;77(8):1143–9.
36. Pagnoux C, Mahr A, Hamidou MA, et al. Azathioprine or methotrexate maintenance for ANCA-associated vasculitis. N Engl J Med 2008;359(26):2790–803.
37. Puechal X, Pagnoux C, Baron G, et al. Adding azathioprine to remission-induction glucocorticoids for eosinophilic granulomatosis with polyangiitis (Churg-Strauss),

microscopic polyangiitis, or polyarteritis nodosa without poor prognosis factors: a randomized, controlled trial. Arthritis Rheumatol 2017;69(11):2175–86.
38. Jones RB, Hiemstra TF, Ballarin J, et al. Mycophenolate mofetil versus cyclophosphamide for remission induction in ANCA-associated vasculitis: a randomised, non-inferiority trial. Ann Rheum Dis 2019;78(3):399–405.
39. Hiemstra TF, Walsh M, Mahr A, et al. Mycophenolate mofetil vs azathioprine for remission maintenance in antineutrophil cytoplasmic antibody-associated vasculitis: a randomized controlled trial. JAMA 2010;304(21):2381–8.
40. Langford CA, Talar-Williams C, Sneller MC. Mycophenolate mofetil for remission maintenance in the treatment of Wegener's granulomatosis. Arthritis Rheum 2004;51(2):278–83.
41. Jayne DR, Gaskin G, Rasmussen N, et al. Randomized trial of plasma exchange or high-dosage methylprednisolone as adjunctive therapy for severe renal vasculitis. J Am Soc Nephrol 2007;18(7):2180–8.
42. Walsh M, Merkel P, Jayne D. The effects of plasma exchange and reduced-dose glucocorticoids during remission-induction for treatment of severe ANCA-associated vasculitis [abstract]. Arthritis Rheumatol 2018;70(suppl 10).
43. Graf J. Central nervous system disease in antineutrophil cytoplasmic antibodies-associated vasculitis. Rheum Dis Clin North Am 2017;43(4):573–8.
44. Fragoulis GE, Lionaki S, Venetsanopoulou A, et al. Central nervous system involvement in patients with granulomatosis with polyangiitis: a single-center retrospective study. Clin Rheumatol 2018;37(3):737–47.
45. Seror R, Mahr A, Ramanoelina J, et al. Central nervous system involvement in Wegener granulomatosis. Medicine 2006;85(1):54–65.
46. Andre R, Cottin V, Saraux JL, et al. Central nervous system involvement in eosinophilic granulomatosis with polyangiitis (Churg-Strauss): report of 26 patients and review of the literature. Autoimmun Rev 2017;16(9):963–9.
47. Lally L, Lebovics RS, Huang WT, et al. Effectiveness of rituximab for the otolaryngologic manifestations of granulomatosis with polyangiitis (Wegener's). Arthritis Care Res 2014;66(9):1403–9.
48. Gopaluni S, Smith RM, Lewin M, et al. Rituximab versus azathioprine as therapy for maintenance of remission for anti-neutrophil cytoplasm antibody-associated vasculitis (RITAZAREM): study protocol for a randomized controlled trial. Trials 2017;18(1):112.
49. Groh M, Pagnoux C, Baldini C, et al. Eosinophilic granulomatosis with polyangiitis (Churg-Strauss) (EGPA) Consensus Task Force recommendations for evaluation and management. Eur J Intern Med 2015;26(7):545–53.
50. Neumann T, Manger B, Schmid M, et al. Cardiac involvement in Churg-Strauss syndrome: impact of endomyocarditis. Medicine 2009;88(4):236–43.
51. Karras A, Pagnoux C, Haubitz M, et al. Randomised controlled trial of prolonged treatment in the remission phase of ANCA-associated vasculitis. Ann Rheum Dis 2017;76(10):1662–8.
52. Guillevin L, Pagnoux C, Karras A, et al. Rituximab versus azathioprine for maintenance in ANCA-associated vasculitis. N Engl J Med 2014;371(19):1771–80.

Is There a Place for Hematopoietic Stem Cell Transplantation in Rheumatology?

Julia Spierings, MD*, Jacob M. van Laar, MD, PhD

KEYWORDS

- Hematopoietic stem cell transplantation • Autoimmune diseases
- Rheumatic diseases • Cell therapy

KEY POINTS

- Hematopoietic stem cell transplantation (HSCT) is increasingly performed in diffuse cutaneous systemic sclerosis.
- Autologous HSCT is indicated in patients with early, poor-prognosis diffuse cutaneous systemic sclerosis and may be considered in patients with other severe, refractory rheumatic diseases if the intended benefits outweigh the risks associated with end-stage organ or joint damage.
- Mortality rates of HSCT have decreased over the years, yet the risks of severe complications associated with HSCT are considerable and have to be weighed against the intended benefits.

INTRODUCTION

Until now, more than 2600 patients with autoimmune diseases have been treated with hematopoietic stem cell transplantation (HSCT).[1,2] Although HSCT is a treatment that carries risks, it may lead to long-term disease-free and even medication-free remission. However, numerous new synthetic and biological agents targeting cytokines or lymphocyte receptors have been developed, which can improve the outcomes of patients with rheumatoid arthritis (RA), juvenile idiopathic arthritis (JIA), and connective tissue diseases (CTDs). With these alternative options available for treatment of rheumatic diseases, one may question if there is still a place for HSCT. In this article, the authors evaluate the experiences with HSCT in rheumatic diseases and discuss its position in modern rheumatology.

Disclosure Statement: No disclosures.
Department of Rheumatology and Clinical Immunology, University Medical Center Utrecht, Heidelberglaan 100, Utrecht 3584 CX, the Netherlands
* Corresponding author.
E-mail address: J.Spierings@umcutrecht.nl

Rheum Dis Clin N Am 45 (2019) 399–416
https://doi.org/10.1016/j.rdc.2019.04.003 rheumatic.theclinics.com
0889-857X/19/

TREATMENT PROCEDURE

HSCT consists of several steps: mobilization of stem cells with chemotherapy and growth-factor, collection of stem cells via leukapheresis, conditioning using myeloablative or lymphoablative chemo(radio)therapy, and reinfusion of stem cells (**Fig. 1**). A variety of treatment regimens have been used for HSCT in rheumatic diseases and, due to the overall small sample sizes of the individual studies, comparison between these studies is difficult. Thus, the optimal HSCT regimen has not yet been established. In general, cyclophosphamide (CYC) is used for mobilization. After the administration of CYC, granulocyte colony-stimulating factor is used to stimulate migration of stem cells from bone marrow so they can be harvested from blood.

Conditioning regimens in HSCT can be myeloablative or nonmyeloablative and vary from high-intensive, including total body irradiation (TBI) or high-dose busulphan; intermediate-intensive, antithymocyte globulin (ATG) combined with either high-dose CYC or other chemotherapeutic drugs; or low-intensive, based on CYC, melphalan, or fludarabine. Nonmyeloablative schemes are most commonly used in autoimmune diseases.

In most studies and trials the reinfused stem cells were autologous, given the higher level of risks associated with allogenic HSCT.[2,3] Graft manipulation by ex vivo selection of CD34 + stem cells remains a matter of debate. Preclinical studies in rodent models of autoimmune disease pointed to the risk of graft contamination with autoreactive T cells. Although CD34 + stem cells are broadly used in clinical practice, there currently is no evidence of their superiority to use of an unselected graft, in terms of rate of duration of remission.[4]

RATIONALE FOR HEMATOPOIETIC STEM CELL TRANSPLANTATION

HSCT aims to reset the immune system into a self-tolerant state.[5] Eradication of autoreactive cells (including memory cells) and reconfiguration of the immune system are induced by the conditioning regimen and reinfusion of hematopoietic stem cells. Depletion of autoreactive T- and B cells by immunoablation drives expansion of the remaining peripheral lymphocyte populations, which is reflected by the reported increase in T-cell receptor oligoclonality.[6–9] In studies performed in systemic sclerosis (SSc) and JIA, an increase or normalization in T-cell receptor repertoire was seen in patients who responded well to HSCT.[7,8,10] In nonresponders, an increase in effector T cells and relatively low numbers of T- and B-regulatory cells were observed following HSCT.[7,8] In patients with systemic lupus erythematosus (SLE), a shift from predominant phenotypic memory B cells toward naïve B cells was seen, while peripheral blood plasmablasts were decreased.[11,12] Furthermore, a marked reduction of immune complex deposition in renal rebiopsies was observed after HSCT.[13] A decline in serum autoantibody titers following HSCT was also detected in several studies and was associated with treatment response.[8,13–15] Taken together, these data highlight the close temporal relationship between restoration of immune balance and clinical responses as a precondition for the development of immune tolerance.[6,13,16–18]

CLINICAL EXPERIENCE IN RHEUMATIC CONDITIONS

Since the mid-90s, HSCT has been used in several rheumatic diseases. The largest cohort studies are those from the European Society for Blood and Marrow Transplantation (EBMT) and the American Society for Blood and Bone Marrow Transplantation/Center for International Blood and Marrow Transplant Research. These cohorts have captured data on patient characteristics and clinical outcome data. In the EBMT

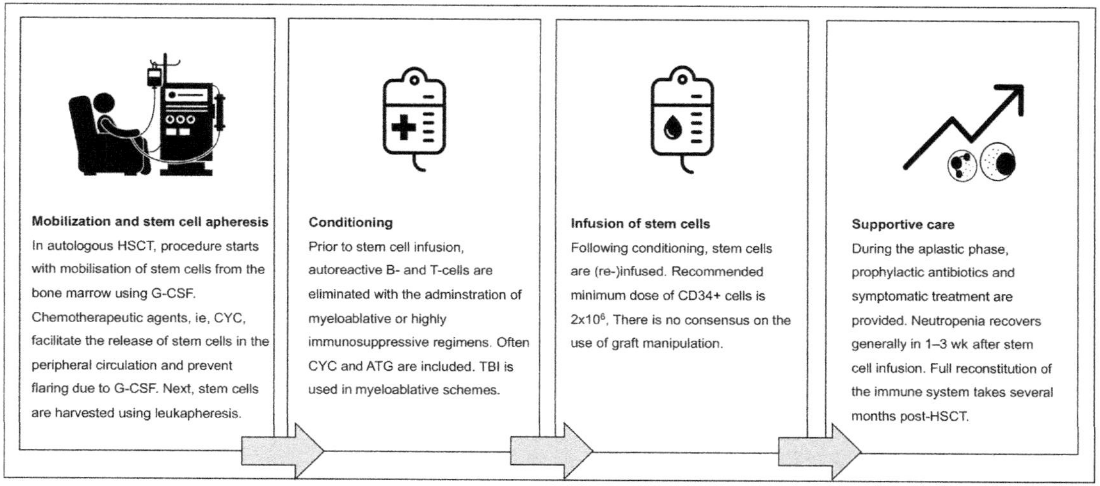
Mobilization and stem cell apheresis
In autologous HSCT, procedure starts with mobilisation of stem cells from the bone marrow using G-CSF. Chemotherapeutic agents, ie, CYC, facilitate the release of stem cells in the peripheral circulation and prevent flaring due to G-CSF. Next, stem cells are harvested using leukapheresis.
Conditioning
Prior to stem cell infusion, autoreactive B- and T-cells are eliminated with the adminstration of myeloablative or highly immunosuppressive regimens. Often CYC and ATG are included. TBI is used in myeloablative schemes.
Infusion of stem cells
Following conditioning, stem cells are (re-)infused. Recommended minimum dose of CD34+ cells is 2x10⁶, There is no consensus on the use of graft manipulation.
Supportive care
During the aplastic phase, prophylactic antibiotics and symptomatic treatment are provided. Neutropenia recovers generally in 1–3 wk after stem cell infusion. Full reconstitution of the immune system takes several months post-HSCT.

Fig. 1. Steps in the HSCT procedure. ATG, antithymocyte globulin; CYC, cyclophosphamide; G-CSF, granulocyte colony-stimulating factor; TBI, total body irradiation.

registry, more than 900 transplant procedures in 247 centers in 40 countries in patients with rheumatic conditions have been registered over the last 20 years.[1] The largest group of patients had a CTD (n = 699), mostly SSc (n = 540) or SLE (n = 108). Other rheumatologic indications were inflammatory arthritis (IA) (n = 166) and vasculitis (n = 45). The annual number of HSCTs performed is increasing, mainly due to the increase in HSCT in SSc, whereas the number of HSCT in SLE and IA continues to drop.[19] Most HSCTs in the EBMT registry involved autologous procedures; only 6% were allogenic, of which the majority were performed in children. Outcomes were significantly better in centers with more experience in HSCT (in number and years). Over time (2000–2004, 2005–2010, and 2011–2015) 3-year outcomes improved as well, among patients undergoing autologous HSCT with intermediate intensity conditioning schemes. The type of autoimmune disease also influenced outcome. SSc was associated with poor outcomes compared with other nonrheumatic autoimmune diseases, such as multiple sclerosis (MS) and Crohn disease (CD).

Clinical Experience in Systemic Sclerosis

SSc is a connective tissue disorder involving systemic inflammation, vascular lesions, and fibrosis.[20] These processes result in skin thickening and organ dysfunction, mainly involving the heart, lungs, and gastrointestinal tract. The diffuse cutaneous clinical subset (diffuse cutaneous SSc [dcSSc]) is characterized by extensive and progressive skin and organ involvement, and a specific autoantibody profile (topoisomerase, RNPIII). Especially in dcSSc, mortality is high, with a 5-year mortality rate of at least 30%.[21] dcSSc is the only rheumatic condition in which HSCT has been used with increased frequency over the last 5 years, and this can be accounted for by the accumulation of evidence of the beneficial effects of HSCT, the lack of equally effective alternative treatments for this disease, and the incorporation of HSCT into national and international treatment guidelines.[4,22,23] Data provided by the European and American registries include overall 3-year survival rates of around 80% and 5-year progression-free survival of 55% (for a detailed overview, see **Table 1**).[2,24] Several phase I and II open-label studies showed that HSCT improved clinical outcomes, such as the modified Rodnan skin score, pulmonary function, and quality of life.[25–27] Superiority of HSCT over intravenous CYC in patients with progressive dcSSc was demonstrated in the 3 controlled, randomized trials published to date.[28–30] The first study, a single-center study (American Scleroderma Stem cell versus Immune Suppression Trial) in 19 patients, showed that autologous HSCT induced regression of both skin and lung fibrosis.[30] The largest, multicenter, open-label phase III Autologous Stem Cell Transplantation International Scleroderma (ASTIS) trial compared monthly intravenous CYC for 1 year with autologous HSCT, using an intermediate intensity conditioning scheme containing CYC and ATG and CD34-selected stem cells in 156 patients with early dcSSc.[28] ASTIS demonstrated better survival rates in the HSCT group after 10 years of follow-up, despite an increased treatment-related mortality (TRM) of 10% during the first year of treatment. The multicenter Scleroderma Cyclophosphamide Or Transplantation (SCOT) trial in 79 patients confirmed superiority of HSCT over CYC after 54 months of follow-up.[29] In contrast to the ASTIS trial, a myeloablative conditioning regimen was used in the SCOT trial with total body irradiation (TBI) and reduced dosages of CYC.

Clinical Experience in Inflammatory Arthritis

Several centers have performed autologous and even allogenic HSCT in patients with RA and refractory JIA.

Table 1
Overview of randomized controlled trials and large cohorts in systemic sclerosis

	N	Characteristics HSCT protocol	Disease Duration Mean, Months	P/EFS (%)	Relapse (%)	TRM (%)	OS (%)	Follow-up Mean, Years
ASSIST, 2011 Phase I trial[30]	10 9	Mob: CYC 2 g/m^2, G-CSF, Con: CYC 200 mg/kg + ATG, HSCT: autologous Control: CYC IV 1 g/m^2, 6 monthly	14 (2–33) 18 (6–36)	80% 2.6 y 13%		0% 0%	100% 100%	2.6
ASTIS, 2014 RCT[28]	79 77	Mob: CYC 4 g/m^2, G-CSF, Con: CYC 200 mg/kg + ATG CD34 + selection, HSCT: autologous Control: CYC IV 750 mg/m^2, 12 monthly	17 18	81% 5.8 y	22% 44%	10%	76% 5.8 y	5.8
SCOT, 2018 RCT[29]	36 39	Mob: G-CSF, Con: CYC 120 mg/kg + ATG, CD34 + selection, TBI: yes, HSCT: autologous Control: CYC750 mg/m^2 IV, 12 monthly	25 29	79% 4.5 y 50%	9% 44%	3% 0%	86% 51%	4.5
EBMT registry, 1996–2007[24]	175	Variable HSCT: autologous	30 (3–256)	63% 3 y		6%	80% 3 y	2.8 (0–9.2)
CIBMTR registry, 1996–2009[2]	85 15	Variable HSCT: autologous HSCT: allogenic	36 (6–64) 31 (10–61)	NR NR	NR NR	6% 27%	83% 3 y 60% 1 y	2.6 (0–12) 1.3 (0–5)

Abbreviations: ASSIST, American Scleroderma Stem cell versus Immune Suppression Trial; ASTIS, Autologous Stem cell Transplantation International Scleroderma trial; ATG, antithymocyte globulin; CIBMTR, Center For International Blood And Marrow Transplant Research; con, conditioning regimen; G-CSF, Granulocyte-colony stimulating factor; IV, intravenous; m, months; Mob, mobilization regimen; NR, not reported; OS, overall survival; P/EFS, progression-/event-free survival without mortality, relapse, or progression of the disease; RCT, randomized controlled trial; SCOT, scleroderma cyclophosphamide or transplantation; TBI, total body irradiation; TRM, treatment-related mortality; y, years.

The prevalence of JIA ranges between 1.6 and 23 per 100,000 children.[31] Children with polyarticular or systemic JIA in particular have a higher risk of developing disease progression.[32] Although no randomized trials have been done in JIA, several observational and phase I/II studies have been published, mostly involving autologous HSCT (an overview is provided in **Table 2**). A retrospective analysis from the EBMT registry included 34 patients with JIA with a mean follow-up time of 29 months.[33] Drug-free complete remission was achieved in 53% of patients and 18% showed a partial response. Complications reported were most often infections. Three patients died of macrophage activation syndrome (MAS); TRM was 9%. In a prospective cohort, 22 patients with systemic or polyarticular JIA were followed during a median period of 80 months after autologous HSCT.[34] Two patients died shortly after treatment due to MAS. Complete remission was achieved in 9 patients (40%), 8 (35%) had a partial response, and 6 experienced a relapse of disease. Two patients died shortly after reintroduction of immunosuppressive medication. In another small study that included 7 patients with JIA who received autologous HSCT, 4 patients experienced medication-free complete remission during a follow-up period of 5 to 8 years, 2 patients relapsed, and 1 died 4 months after HSCT.[35] Two patients had a relapse within 1 year after HSCT. A retrospective analysis of allogenic HSCT using a reduced intensity conditioning regimen containing alemtuzumab and fludarabine showed good effects.[36] This study included 7 systemic and 5 patients with polyarticular JIA who were refractory to standard therapy or even to autologous HSCT. After a mean follow-up of 29 months, all patients experienced significant improvement of arthritis and MAS. Eleven patients achieved drug-free remission. Three patients developed acute graft-versus-host disease (GvHD). The incidence of infections following HSCT was high: half of all patients experienced viral infections or reactivation, 4 patients experienced bacterial infections, and 1 patient developed a severe fungal infection. Two patients died as complications of treatment. Thus, although the results from these studies showed improvement of disease activity and quality of life, the procedure carried significant risks of infectious complications. In RA, mostly autologous HSCT is performed. In the EBMT registry, overall 5-year survival rate was 94% among 76 patients with RA.[37] Although the 5-year progression-free survival rate was low (18%), there was a partial response in 67% (American College of Rheumatology 50 response). Patients with seronegative RA ($n = 11$) had a significantly better response than those with seropositive disease ($P = .02$). No TRM was reported. In a small study including 14 patients with refractory RA, 7 patients relapsed after HSCT.[38] Reintroduction of disease-modifying antirheumatic drugs (DMARDs) resulted in sustained disease control in 3 patients, even with DMARDs that were previously ineffective in these individuals. Response was associated with the persistence of serum autoantibodies and inflammatory changes in the synovium.[39]

Australian investigators performed autologous HSCT in 33 patients with refractory RA.[40] Patients were randomly allocated to receive CD34 + selected cells or an unmanipulated graft. Although no serious side effects were reported, treatment response was disappointing in both arms, with a relapse in the first year after HSCT occurring in 73%. There was no benefit observed in the group that received CD34 + cells compared with the group that received unmanipulated cells. Another report of 2 patients receiving syngeneic HSCT described each as having a partial remission after 28 and 70 months.[3] There has been one report of allogenic HSCT with complete remission after 45 months. However, since the introduction of effective biological agents, HSCT has become uncommon in patients with JIA or RA.[19]

Table 2
Overview of studies in inflammatory arthritis

	N	Characteristics HSCT Protocol	Disease Duration Mean, Months	P/EFS (%)	Relapse (%)	TRM (%)	OS (%)	Follow-up Mean, Years
JIA								
EBMT registry 1996–2007[24]	65	Variable HSCT: autologous	74 m (11–233)	52 (3y)	NR	11%	82% 3 y	5.6 y (0.5–9)
Brinkman et al,[34] 2007 Prospective cohort	22	Con: CYC (200 mg/kg), ATG (20 mg/kg), CD34 + selection and TBI (4Gy). HSCT: autologous	70 m (13–135)	40%	23%	9%	91%	6.7 y
Abinun et al,[35] 2009 Retrospective cohort	7	Con: different agents and dosages, CD34 1 selection. HSCT: autologous	NR	57% (5–8 y)	22%	14%	86%	6.5 y
Silva et al,[36] 2018 Retrospective cohort	16	Con: fludarabine (150 mg/m^2), melphalan (140 mg/m^2), alemtuzumab (1.0 mg/kg). CD34 1 selection. HSCT: allogenic	79 m	78%	19%	13%	87%	2.4 y
RA								
Verburg et al,[38] 2001, Open label phase I/II study	14	Mob: CYC 4 mg/m^2, G-CSF, Con: CYC 200 mg/kg, CD34 + selection. HSCT: autologous	120 m	17% ACR70,1.2 y	58%	0%	100%	0.6–1.8 y
Moore et al,[40] 2002, RCT	33	Mob: CYC 200 mg/kg, G-CSF, Con: CYC (high dose), HSCT: autologous CD34 + selection: yes no	120 m (2–19 y)	ACR70, 1 y 28% 53%	87%	0%	100%, 1 y	1 y
EBMT registry 1996–2007[3,24]	89 3	Variable HSCT: autologous HSCT: allogenic	86 m (21–284) NR	23% (3 y) 33% (3 y)	NR 67%	1% 0%	98%, 3 y 100%, 3 y	2.3 y (0.5–9) 4 y (2–5.8)

Abbreviations: ACR, American College of Rheumatology; ATG, antithymocyte globulin; CIBMTR, Center for International Blood and Marrow Transplant Research; m, months; Mob, mobilization; NR, not reported; OS, overall survival; P/EFS, progression-/event-free survival without mortality, relapse, or progression of the disease; RCT, randomized controlled trial; y, years.

Clinical Experience in Systemic Lupus Erythematosus

SLE is a heterogeneous systemic autoimmune disorder associated with severe multi-organ involvement. Despite immunosuppressive treatment, organ damage develops in 32% to 42% of patients.[41,42] Since the first case report of a successful autologous HSCT was published, approximately 300 patients with SLE worldwide have undergone HSCT.[43]

In data from the EBMT registry (collected between 1995 and 2002), the overall survival rate was 76% in 53 patients with SLE (median disease duration was 59 months, median age 29 years, 62% lupus nephritis) with a progression-free survival of 52% after 5 years[44]; TRM was 12%. Causes of death were gastrointestinal hemorrhage (n = 1), infection (n = 3), thrombotic thrombocytopenic purpura (n = 1), and secondary leukemia (n = 1). Relapse was observed in 32% after 6 months post-HSCT. No difference in relapse rate was observed between groups receiving unselected or CD34-selected stem cells. Interestingly, in an analysis of the EMBT registry in patients with SLE included from 2001 until 2008, outcomes were significantly better in patients who received CD34-selected stem cells compared with unselected cells.[45] Yet, this difference could also be attributed to a difference in conditioning schemes.

A prospective cohort (n = 24) from China observed decreased SLE Disease Activity Index scores following HSCT.[11] Compared with the other studies in SLE, the event-free survival rate was much higher (86%), after a median follow-up period of 120 months. Proteinuria improved significantly in the 15 patients suffering lupus nephritis. TRM was 4% (n = 2) and 46% flared. Hydroxychloroquine therapy was maintained in 60% of patients after HSCT. Flare treatment included low-dose methotrexate and mycophenolate mofetil. Another prospective Chinese study (n = 22) also showed improvement of proteinuria, an overall survival rate after 5 years of 95%, and a 5-year event-free survival rate of 68%.[13] There were no treatment-related deaths. The importance of choosing the optimal conditioning regimen was emphasized by a recently published study with 2 different conditioning regimens in autologous HSCT. CYC was combined either with the conventional rabbit ATG (n = 26) or with alemtuzumab (n = 4); rituximab was added in both arms. Because graft manipulation was not possible (CD34 selection columns from American manufacturers were not available), it was hypothesized that in vivo alemtuzumab would remove autoreactive T cells. However, none of the 4 patients in this treatment arm reached remission and even 2 patients died due to disease progression.[46]

Among children with SLE, few cases of HSCT have been reported in the literature. In the EMBT registry, 17 patients with pediatric SLE were included.[44] These patients all received autologous using conditioning regimens containing CYC, ATG, or TBI. Complete remission was achieved in half of all patients after a follow-up period of 26 months. TRM was 7% (n = 1). A report of 2 other cases showed variable results as well.[47] Over the long term, a relevant issue in treating young patients with HSCT is fertility and pregnancy. One observational study followed 15 SLE patients who received autologous HSCT with a conditioning regimen including CYC and ATG, for a mean period of 12 years (2–16 years).[48] Four female patients, who experienced sustained clinical remission after HSCT, had 5 pregnancies and 6 healthy children during follow-up. There were no miscarriages. Allogenic HSCT is performed less often in SLE. A retrospective Indian study presented the results of 27 patients with SLE treated with nonmyeloablative, low-intensity conditioning (CYC, ATG, and steroids) followed by allogenic HSCT (mean follow-up period was 57 months).[49] The mean disease-free period was 7 months (2–13 months). No severe complications, such as GvHD, were reported; this is quite unusual, especially in allogenic HSCT. In a case series of 3 patients, more sustainable benefit was observed with follow-up duration up to 6 years.[50] A systematic review of the literature yielded 25 studies of HSCT that included 279 patients with SLE.[51] All studies showed a decrease in disease activity and overall survival. Pooled analysis showed an overall mortality of 8%, although heterogeneity between studies was high ($I^2 = 87\%$). In this review, 44 patients with SLE had secondary antiphospholipid syndrome. Post-HSCT, anticoagulation could be discontinued in 73% of patients without thrombotic complications during follow-up (8–28 months). In 9% (n = 5) of patients, antiphospholipid antibodies were not detectable after treatment.[52]

CLINICAL EXPERIENCE IN OTHER RHEUMATIC CONDITIONS

Less data are available on HSCT in other rheumatic diseases. From the EBMT registry, a retrospective analysis of 15 patients with several types of vasculitis (granulomatosis with polyangiitis, eosinophilic granulomatosis with polyangiitis, cryoglobulinemia, polychondritis, polyarteritis nodosa, Takayasu arteritis, Behçet disease [BD]) showed complete remission in 46% (n = 12) and partial remission in 46% of patients following autologous HSCT.[53] Mean follow-up duration was 45 months and the overall survival rate was 80%. TRM was 7% (n = 1) due to GvHD. In addition to the 3 cases of BD included in the EBMT registry, a systematic review described HSCT in 20 patients with BD.[54] Eleven had concomitant hematological conditions and 9 refractory BD. In the patients with BD, 8 received autologous HSCT, of whom 80% experienced improvement of neurologic and gastrointestinal symptoms and even diminution of vascular lesions. The BD patients with hematological conditions had gastrointestinal involvement. After HSCT, which was allogenic in most cases, intestinal ulcers resolved and all patients experienced improvement of gastrointestinal symptoms. One patient developed grade-4 GvHD and one patient died of infectious disease.

SAFETY OF HEMATOPOIETIC STEM CELL TRANSPLANTATION

HSCT in autoimmune disease is associated with considerable morbidity and related mortality. In the EMBT registry, 100-day TRM was 5% (95% confidence interval [CI]: 3%–7%) in all patients with autoimmune diseases treated with HSCT.[24] The most common complication of HSCT is infection, due to the use of intense immunosuppressive medication before and during the HSCT procedure.[4] Because of neutropenia early in the procedure, bacterial or fungal infections can occur. Prolonged lymphopenia may lead to reactivation of latent viruses and opportunistic infections. The introduction of prophylactic broad-spectrum antibacterial, antifungal, and antiviral prophylaxis for at least 100 days after transplantation has reduced the risk of these complications.[4,55] In general, long-term complications of HSCT include endocrine dysfunction, infertility, autoimmunity, renal dysfunction, and malignancies.[32,56] In patients with autoimmune diseases who underwent HSCT, the long-term risk of developing solid tumors was twice as high in comparison with the general population.[2,24]

Toxicity and risk of TRM varies depending on the choice of donor cells.[19] Compared with autologous HSCT, allogenic HSCT had a higher risk of death (30%–42% 1 year post-HSCT), particularly because of the occurrence of GvHD after allogenic HSCT. Severity of the underlying disease may have contributed to the high mortality rate after allogenic HSCT in patients with autoimmune disease. The occurrence of adverse effects is also associated with the conditioning regimen used.[19] Studies reporting on HSCT used different protocols (see **Tables 1** and **2**; **Table 3**) and only one study compared different regimens directly.[46] The use of TBI increases the risk of

Table 3
Overview of hematopoietic stem cell transplantation studies in systemic lupus erythematosus

	N	Characteristics Treatment Protocol	Disease Duration Mean, Months	P/EFS (%)	Relapse (%)	TRM (%)	OS (%)	Follow-up Mean, Years
EBMT registry 1995–2002[44]	53	Variable HSCT: autologous	59 m	52%	32%, 6 m	12	76%	5 y
EBMT registry 1996–2007[3,24]	85 2	Variable HSCT: autologous HSCT: allogenic	58 m (2–396 m)	54%, 3 y	32%, 6 m	6 50	87%, 3 y 50%, 3 y	2 y (2–10) 1.8 y (0–3)
CIBMTR registry 1996–2005[73]	50	Mob: CYC 2 g/m^2, G-CSF, Con: CYC 200 mg/kg, ATG CD34 + selection. HSCT: autologous	NR	50%, 5 y	NR	4	84% ,5 y	2.5 y (0.5–7.5)
Vanikar et al,[49] 2007 Retrospective cohort	27	CsA 5mg/kg, steroids, ATG HSCT: allogenic Post-HSCT; steroids	21 m (9–41)	NR	NR	0%	100%	4.9 y (4.2–5.4)
Leng et al,[11] 2017 Prospective cohort	24	Mob: CYC 2 g/m^2, G-CSF, Con: CYC 200 mg/kg, TBI or ATG. CD34 + selection. HSCT: autologous	60 m (14–192 m)	86%, 10 y	46%	4%	86%, 10 y	10 y
Burt et al,[46] 2018 Prospective cohort	26 4	Mob: CYC 2 g/m^2, G-CSF. Con: 1. CYC 200 mg/kg, ATG, RTX 2. CYC 200 mg/kg, alemtuzumab 60 mg, RTX (500 mg) HSCT: autologous Post-HSCT; HCQ	10.5 y (1–33)	62%, 5 y 0%, 5 y	38%, 5 y -	0% 0%	100%, 5 y 50%, 5 y	5 y
Cao et al,[13] 2018 Prospective cohort	22	Mob: CYC 2–4 g/m^2, G-CSF, Con: CYC (200 mg/kg), ATG, steroids. TBI (n = 1), RTX in one patient. CD34 + selection, HSCT: autologous	NR	68%, 5 y 53%, 10 y	42%	0%	95%, 5 y	9.4 y (4.3–12.3)

Abbreviations: CIBMTR, Center for International Blood and Marrow Transplant Research; CsA, cyclosporine A; HCQ, hydroxychloroquine; m, months; Mob, mobilization; NR, not reported; OS, overall survival; P/EFS, progression-/event-free survival without mortality, relapse, or progression of the disease; RCT, randomized controlled trial; RTX, rituximab; y, years.

malignancies on the long term. However, using a myeloablative regimen including TBI, in order to eliminate autoreactive clones, may limit the CYC dose, which can be toxic as well at high doses, especially in SSc.[29] Heterogeneity between studies complicates comparison of conditioning regimens, thus no clear statements can be made about the safest regimen.

Complications seemed more often in HSCT in SSc, compared with CD or MS or other rheumatic conditions.[17] This might be explained by the presence of involvement of vital organs, such as the heart, lungs, or kidney, which make patients more vulnerable to cardiotoxic agents, infections, and sepsis.[57–59] Especially in patients with compromised cardiac function, complications can occur due to the higher cardiac demand during transplant-related fever, neutropenic infection, and volume overload by infusion. Therefore, performing HSCT early in disease course could prevent some of these adverse events when organ involvement is limited. TRM in studies in SSc varied between 3% and 10%.[28,29,60] In both the ASTIS and SCOT trials, smoking status was shown to negatively impact the differences in survival. Apart from the higher rate of treatment-related side effects, disease-related mortality was also high in SSc (13%), which can be explained by the systemic manifestations of the condition.

Lastly, with regard to safety, in some studies, a significant center effect was found with regard to mortality rates, possibly related to routine interdisciplinary collaboration and participation in clinical trials in centers with higher number of HSCT in rheumatic diseases.[61] To optimize safety of the treatment procedure it is key to carefully screen the patient for cardiopulmonary complications or comorbidities. Centralization of HSCT in specialized centers should be considered.[62] Altogether, all elements related to HSCT, such as patient selection, cardiopulmonary screening, timing of treatment, treatment procedures, and supportive care, are key to treat patients with HSCT successfully and safely. Importantly, this requires close collaboration of a multidisciplinary team of experienced clinicians.

ECONOMIC ASPECTS OF NOVEL THERAPIES AND HEMATOPOIETIC STEM CELL TRANSPLANTATION

The impact of chronic rheumatic autoimmune diseases on society is far from negligible, especially in the group of patients eligible for HSCT.[63,64] Although this group is relatively small, health care consumption by this seriously ill population is significant.[65] Moreover, participation in the workforce is often limited due to the disease and treatment. Health care costs are a concern worldwide, especially with regard to new agents and complex procedures in patients with chronic conditions. HSCT is a complex and expensive treatment, costing approximately USD $100,000 to 150,000.[66–68] Biologics and other new targeted therapies are expensive too, and unfortunately, they require long-term use and are not universally effective. A drug-free remission outcome of HSCT may lead to significant cost savings on the long run.[69] Irrespective of the possible economic benefits, complications emerging from chronic immunosuppressive medication can be avoided by HSCT. One exploratory cost-effectiveness analysis showed that HSCT might be cost-effective in MS in some situations.[70] Relapse rates were included in this analysis. No cost-effectiveness studies of HSCT in rheumatic conditions have been performed.

DISCUSSION

Despite the wide use of new treatments, such as biologics, autologous HSCT is increasingly performed worldwide in rheumatic conditions. Outcomes including survival have improved over the years due to growing experience and optimized supportive care. In **Box 1** an overview of the indications for HSCT is shown.

A key challenge in daily practice is making the actual decision to pursue with HSCT and planning for it. With regard to optimal timing of HSCT in the course of rheumatic diseases, it may seem preferable to evaluate a patient's response to immunosuppressive therapy first, before proceeding to HSCT, because conventional immunosuppressive therapies are associated with fewer adverse events. On the other hand, in the time frame needed to evaluate the effects of the initiated therapy, disease progression could evolve beyond the point of eligibility for HSCT. Moreover, HSCT may be less effective in patients with advanced organ damage and enduring immune dysregulation. Because there are no specific guidelines on patient selection and timing, the treatment choice lies primarily with the patient and his or her physician and largely depends on the patients' preferences. From a patients' perspective, both this decision and treatment have a huge impact on their personal life. Clinicians should provide clear information adjusted to the individual and support the decision-making process by weighing the pros and cons of HSCT together with the patient.[71] An argument in favor of HSCT is the accumulating evidence of the beneficial effects of HSCT. Particularly in progressive dcSSc, the decision to opt for HSCT is supported by the results of 3 randomized controlled trials that compared HSCT with treatment with CYC. Still, treatment regimens and guidelines for patient selection should be optimized in order to

Box 1
The place of autologous hematopoietic stem cell transplantation in rheumatic diseases

Diagnosis	Position of HSCT	Evidence
Diffuse cutaneous systemic sclerosis	HSCT is indicated in: • Acute onset of disease, rapid progression • Short disease duration	Beneficial effects confirmed in clinical trials.
Systemic lupus erythematosus	HSCT is an option in • Refractory disease to conventional therapy (CYC, MMF) • Short disease duration	Observational studies show promising results. Clinical trials ongoing.
Juvenile chronic arthritis and rheumatoid arthritis	HSCT is an option in • Severe disease with persistent activity • Refractory to several combinations of DMARDs including biologics	Observational studies show reasonable effects and risks. No data from controlled clinical trials available or ongoing.
Other rheumatic conditions[a]	HSCT could be an option in • Severe and refractory disease	Only data available from case-reports or case-series.

Conditions: close multidisciplinary collaboration in patient selection, treatment, and follow-up; treatment in specialized and experienced centers; early referral of patients to an expert center to achieve the best clinical effects of treatment; preferably, inclusion of HSCT patients in clinical trials.

Abbreviation: MMF, mycophenolate mofetil.

[a] Vasculitis, Behçet disease, antiphospholipid syndrome, Sjogren syndrome, psoriatic arthritis.

decrease the number of severe complications. Small sample sizes and heterogeneity between studies with regard to treatment regimens, patient selection, and definitions on remission and other outcomes complicate comparison of current available data.

In contrast to dcSSc, the need for HSCT in other rheumatic diseases, such as SLE and IA, has declined, as biologics and other new therapies have shown to be effective and well tolerated in most patients. Even so, especially in SLE, there is encouraging evidence that HSCT could be beneficial in selected patients. At the moment, there are 2 trials ongoing in SLE (NCT00750971, NCT00325741). In RA, in the absence of large randomized trials, a Markov clinical decision analysis was done to compare effects of HSCT and conventional therapy.[72] The model predicted that HSCT would be superior to conventional treatment if TRM remained low (<3.3%) or if treatment effects are sustained for 5 years. Although performed early in the biologics era, these analyses suggest that selected patients with RA could indeed benefit from HSCT. The small differences in quality-adjusted life years between patients treated with HSCT and conventional therapy in this model also highlights the important role that the patient should play in the treatment decision. Another concern about HSCT is the substantial relapse rate. Factors contributing to relapse could be conditioning regimens, use of graft manipulation, or timing of HSCT in the disease course. Flares following HSCT seem more amenable to treatment with conventional immunosuppressive agents. However, the benefits of routine maintenance therapy following HSCT have to be investigated.

The remaining challenge and probably the main reason to be reluctant to perform HSCT is the relatively high rate of complications related to the therapy. However, safety has improved over the years. In some cases, HSCT might be the only effective treatment available and thus could therefore make these risks acceptable. Yet, the decision to pursue this treatment depends on the personal preferences of the individual patient and should be discussed carefully. In addition, economical aspects of HSCT compared with other treatments should be included in the discussion about the role of HSCT in treating rheumatic conditions. Unfortunately, cost-effectiveness studies are lacking.

Based on the available evidence, autologous HSCT may be considered in patients with severe and refractory rheumatic disease, particularly those with poor-prognosis early dcSSc. Future research should focus on the optimal selection of patients who are most likely to benefit from HSCT, timing in the course of the disease, optimal effective and safe conditioning regimens and post-transplantation management, and economic aspects.

REFERENCES

1. Snowden JA, Sharrack B, Akil M, et al. Autologous haematopoietic stem cell transplantation (aHSCT) for severe resistant autoimmune and inflammatory diseases - a guide for the generalist. Clin Med (Lond) 2018;18(4):329–34.
2. Pasquini MC, Voltarelli J, Atkins HL, et al. Transplantation for autoimmune diseases in north and South America: a report of the Center for International Blood and Marrow Transplant Research. Biol Blood Marrow Transplant 2012;18(10): 1471–8.
3. Daikeler T, Hugle T, Farge D, et al. Allogeneic hematopoietic SCT for patients with autoimmune diseases. Bone Marrow Transplant 2009;44(1):27–33.
4. Snowden JA, Saccardi R, Allez M, et al. Haematopoietic SCT in severe autoimmune diseases: updated guidelines of the European Group for Blood and Marrow Transplantation. Bone Marrow Transplant 2012;47(6):770–90.

5. van Rhijn-Brouwer FCC, Spierings J, van Laar JM. Autologous hematopoietic stem cell transplantation in systemic sclerosis: a reset to tolerance? Immunol Lett 2018;195:88–96.
6. Henes J, Glaeser L, Kotter I, et al. Analysis of anti-topoisomerase I antibodies in patients with systemic sclerosis before and after autologous stem cell transplantation. Rheumatology 2017;56(3):451–6.
7. Arruda LCM, Malmegrim KCR, Lima-Junior JR, et al. Immune rebound associates with a favorable clinical response to autologous HSCT in systemic sclerosis patients. Blood Adv 2018;2(2):126–41.
8. Farge D, Arruda LC, Brigant F, et al. Long-term immune reconstitution and T cell repertoire analysis after autologous hematopoietic stem cell transplantation in systemic sclerosis patients. J Hematol Oncol 2017;10(1):21.
9. Wu Q, Pesenacker AM, Stansfield A, et al. Immunological characteristics and T-cell receptor clonal diversity in children with systemic juvenile idiopathic arthritis undergoing T-cell-depleted autologous stem cell transplantation. Immunology 2014;142(2):227–36.
10. Delemarre EM, van den Broek T, Mijnheer G, et al. Autologous stem cell transplantation aids autoimmune patients by functional renewal and TCR diversification of regulatory T cells. Blood 2016;127(1):91–101.
11. Leng XM, Jiang Y, Zhou DB, et al. Good outcome of severe lupus patients with high-dose immunosuppressive therapy and autologous peripheral blood stem cell transplantation: a 10-year follow-up study. Clin Exp Rheumatol 2017;35(3): 494–9.
12. Alexander T, Thiel A, Rosen O, et al. Depletion of autoreactive immunologic memory followed by autologous hematopoietic stem cell transplantation in patients with refractory SLE induces long-term remission through de novo generation of a juvenile and tolerant immune system. Blood 2009;113(1):214–23.
13. Cao C, Wang M, Sun J, et al. Autologous peripheral blood haematopoietic stem cell transplantation for systemic lupus erythematosus: the observation of long-term outcomes in a Chinese centre. Clin Exp Rheumatol 2017;35(3):500–7.
14. Farge D, Henegar C, Carmagnat M, et al. Analysis of immune reconstitution after autologous bone marrow transplantation in systemic sclerosis. Arthritis Rheum 2005;52(5):1555–63.
15. Bohgaki T, Atsumi T, Bohgaki M, et al. Immunological reconstitution after autologous hematopoietic stem cell transplantation in patients with systemic sclerosis: relationship between clinical benefits and intensity of immunosuppression. J Rheumatol 2009;36(6):1240–8.
16. Muraro PA, Douek DC, Packer A, et al. Thymic output generates a new and diverse TCR repertoire after autologous stem cell transplantation in multiple sclerosis patients. J Exp Med 2005;201(5):805–16.
17. Ponchel F, Verburg RJ, Bingham SJ, et al. Interleukin-7 deficiency in rheumatoid arthritis: consequences for therapy-induced lymphopenia. Arthritis Res Ther 2005;7(1):R80–92.
18. Alexander T, Sattler A, Templin L, et al. Foxp3+ Helios+ regulatory T cells are expanded in active systemic lupus erythematosus. Ann Rheum Dis 2013;72(9): 1549–58.
19. Snowden JA, Badoglio M, Labopin M, et al. Evolution, trends, outcomes, and economics of hematopoietic stem cell transplantation in severe autoimmune diseases. Blood Adv 2017;1(27):2742–55.
20. LeRoy EC, Black C, Fleischmajer R, et al. Scleroderma (systemic sclerosis): classification, subsets and pathogenesis. J Rheumatol 1988;15(2):202–5.

21. Ioannidis JP, Vlachoyiannopoulos PG, Haidich AB, et al. Mortality in systemic sclerosis: an international meta-analysis of individual patient data. Am J Med 2005;118(1):2–10.
22. Kowal-Bielecka O, Fransen J, Avouac J, et al. Update of EULAR recommendations for the treatment of systemic sclerosis. Ann Rheum Dis 2017;76(8):1327–39.
23. Denton CP, Hughes M, Gak N, et al. BSR and BHPR guideline for the treatment of systemic sclerosis. Rheumatology 2016;55(10):1906–10.
24. Farge D, Labopin M, Tyndall A, et al. Autologous hematopoietic stem cell transplantation for autoimmune diseases: an observational study on 12 years' experience from the European Group for Blood and Marrow Transplantation Working Party on Autoimmune Diseases. Haematologica 2010;95(2):284–92.
25. Henes JC, Schmalzing M, Vogel W, et al. Optimization of autologous stem cell transplantation for systemic sclerosis – a single-center longterm experience in 26 patients with severe organ manifestations. J Rheumatol 2012;39(2):269–75.
26. Nash RA, McSweeney PA, Crofford LJ, et al. High-dose immunosuppressive therapy and autologous hematopoietic cell transplantation for severe systemic sclerosis: long-term follow-up of the US multicenter pilot study. Blood 2007;110(4): 1388–96.
27. Del Papa N, Onida F, Zaccara E, et al. Autologous hematopoietic stem cell transplantation has better outcomes than conventional therapies in patients with rapidly progressive systemic sclerosis. Bone Marrow Transplant 2017;52(1):53–8.
28. van Laar JM, Farge D, Sont JK, et al. Autologous hematopoietic stem cell transplantation vs intravenous pulse cyclophosphamide in diffuse cutaneous systemic sclerosis: a randomized clinical trial. JAMA 2014;311(24):2490–8.
29. Sullivan KM, Goldmuntz EA, Keyes-Elstein L, et al. Myeloablative Autologous Stem-Cell Transplantation for Severe Scleroderma. N Engl J Med 2018;378(1): 35–47.
30. Burt RK, Shah SJ, Dill K, et al. Autologous non-myeloablative haemopoietic stem-cell transplantation compared with pulse cyclophosphamide once per month for systemic sclerosis (ASSIST): an open-label, randomised phase 2 trial. Lancet 2011;378(9790):498–506.
31. Thierry S, Fautrel B, Lemelle I, et al. Prevalence and incidence of juvenile idiopathic arthritis: a systematic review. Joint Bone Spine 2014;81(2):112–7.
32. Prince FH, Otten MH, van Suijlekom-Smit LW. Diagnosis and management of juvenile idiopathic arthritis. BMJ 2010;341:c6434.
33. de Kleer I, Vastert B, Klein M, et al. Autologous stem cell transplantation for autoimmunity induces immunologic self-tolerance by reprogramming autoreactive T cells and restoring the CD4+CD25+ immune regulatory network. Blood 2005;107(4):1696–702.
34. Brinkman DM, de Kleer IM, ten Cate R, et al. Autologous stem cell transplantation in children with severe progressive systemic or polyarticular juvenile idiopathic arthritis: long-term follow-up of a prospective clinical trial. Arthritis Rheum 2007; 56(7):2410–21.
35. Abinun M, Flood TJ, Cant AJ, et al. Autologous T cell depleted hematopoietic stem cell transplantation in children with severe juvenile idiopathic arthritis in the UK (2000–2007). Mol Immunol 2009;47(1):46–51.
36. Silva JMF, Ladomenou F, Carpenter B, et al. Allogeneic hematopoietic stem cell transplantation for severe, refractory juvenile idiopathic arthritis. Blood Adv 2018;2(7):777–86.

37. Snowden JA, Passweg J, Moore JJ, et al. Autologous hemopoietic stem cell transplantation in severe rheumatoid arthritis: a report from the EBMT and ABMTR. J Rheumatol 2004;31(3):482–8.
38. Verburg RJ, Kruize AA, van den Hoogen FH, et al. High-dose chemotherapy and autologous hematopoietic stem cell transplantation in patients with rheumatoid arthritis: results of an open study to assess feasibility, safety, and efficacy. Arthritis Rheum 2001;44(4):754–60.
39. van Oosterhout M, Verburg RJ, Levarht EW, et al. High dose chemotherapy and syngeneic stem cell transplantation in a patient with refractory rheumatoid arthritis: poor response associated with persistence of host autoantibodies and synovial abnormalities. Ann Rheum Dis 2005;64(12):1783–5.
40. Moore J, Brooks P, Milliken S, et al. A pilot randomized trial comparing CD34-selected versus unmanipulated hemopoietic stem cell transplantation for severe, refractory rheumatoid arthritis. Arthritis Rheum 2002;46(9):2301–9.
41. Tsang ASMW, Bultink IE, Heslinga M, et al. Both prolonged remission and Lupus Low Disease Activity State are associated with reduced damage accrual in systemic lupus erythematosus. Rheumatology 2017;56(1):121–8.
42. Zen M, Iaccarino L, Gatto M, et al. Prolonged remission in Caucasian patients with SLE: prevalence and outcomes. Ann Rheum Dis 2015;74(12):2117–22.
43. Marmont AM, van Lint MT, Gualandi F, et al. Autologous marrow stem cell transplantation for severe systemic lupus erythematosus of long duration. Lupus 1997; 6(6):545–8.
44. Jayne D, Passweg J, Marmont A, et al. Autologous stem cell transplantation for systemic lupus erythematosus. Lupus 2004;13(3):168–76.
45. Alchi B, Jayne D, Labopin M, et al. Autologous haematopoietic stem cell transplantation for systemic lupus erythematosus: data from the European Group for Blood and Marrow Transplantation registry. Lupus 2013;22(3):245–53.
46. Burt RK, Han X, Gozdziak P, et al. Five year follow-up after autologous peripheral blood hematopoietic stem cell transplantation for refractory, chronic, corticosteroid-dependent systemic lupus erythematosus: effect of conditioning regimen on outcome. Bone Marrow Transplant 2018;53(6):692–700.
47. Chen J, Wang Y, Kunkel G, et al. Use of CD34+ autologous stem cell transplantation in the treatment of children with refractory systemic lupus erythematosus. Clin Rheumatol 2005;24(5):464–8.
48. Massenkeil G, Alexander T, Rosen O, et al. Long-term follow-up of fertility and pregnancy in autoimmune diseases after autologous haematopoietic stem cell transplantation. Rheumatol Int 2016;36(11):1563–8.
49. Vanikar AV, Modi PR, Patel RD, et al. Hematopoietic stem cell transplantation in autoimmune diseases: the Ahmedabad experience. Transplant Proc 2007; 39(3):703–8.
50. Gladstone DE, Petri M, Bolanos-Meade J, et al. Long-term systemic lupus erythematosus disease control after allogeneic bone marrow transplantation. Lupus 2017;26(7):773–6.
51. Leone A, Radin M, Almarzooqi AM, et al. Autologous hematopoietic stem cell transplantation in Systemic Lupus Erythematosus and antiphospholipid syndrome: a systematic review. Autoimmun Rev 2017;16(5):469–77.
52. Statkute L, Traynor A, Oyama Y, et al. Antiphospholipid syndrome in patients with systemic lupus erythematosus treated by autologous hematopoietic stem cell transplantation. Blood 2005;106(8):2700–9.
53. Daikeler T, Kotter I, Bocelli Tyndall C, et al. Haematopoietic stem cell transplantation for vasculitis including Behcet's disease and polychondritis: a retrospective

analysis of patients recorded in the European Bone Marrow Transplantation and European League Against Rheumatism databases and a review of the literature. Ann Rheum Dis 2007;66(2):202–7.
54. Soysal T, Salihoglu A, Esatoglu SN, et al. Bone marrow transplantation for Behcet's disease: a case report and systematic review of the literature. Rheumatology 2014;53(6):1136–41.
55. Daikeler T, Tichelli A, Passweg J. Complications of autologous hematopoietic stem cell transplantation for patients with autoimmune diseases. Pediatr Res 2012;71(4 Pt 2):439–44.
56. Tichelli A, Rovo A, Passweg J, et al. Late complications after hematopoietic stem cell transplantation. Expert Rev Hematol 2009;2(5):583–601.
57. van Laar JM, Farge D, Tyndall A, et al. Cardiac assessment before stem cell transplantation for systemic sclerosis—reply. JAMA 2017;312(17):1803–4.
58. Spierings J, van Rhijn-Brouwer FCC, van Laar JM. Hematopoietic stem-cell transplantation in systemic sclerosis: an update. Curr Opin Rheumatol 2018;30(6): 541–7.
59. Burt R, Shah SJ, Gheorghiade M, et al. Hematopoietic stem cell transplantation for systemic sclerosis: if you are confused, remember: "it is a matter of the heart". J Rheumatol 2012;39(2):206–9.
60. Farge D, Gluckman E. Autologous HSCT in systemic sclerosis: a step forward. Lancet 2011;378(9790):460–2.
61. Alexander T, Farge D, Badoglio M, et al. Hematopoietic stem cell therapy for autoimmune diseases - Clinical experience and mechanisms. J Autoimmun 2018;92:35–46.
62. Farge D, Burt RK, Oliveira MC, et al. Cardiopulmonary assessment of patients with systemic sclerosis for hematopoietic stem cell transplantation: recommendations from the European Society for Blood and Marrow Transplantation Autoimmune Diseases Working Party and collaborating partners. Bone Marrow Transplant 2017;52(11):1495–503.
63. Villaverde-Hueso A, Sanchez-Valle E, Alvarez E, et al. Estimating the burden of scleroderma disease in Spain. J Rheumatol 2007;34(11):2236–42.
64. Chevreul K, Brigham KB, Gandre C, et al. The economic burden and health-related quality of life associated with systemic sclerosis in France. Scand J Rheumatol 2015;44(3):238–46.
65. Meijs J, Zirkzee EJ, Schouffoer AA, et al. Health-care utilization in Dutch systemic sclerosis patients. Clin Rheumatol 2013;33(6):825–32.
66. Sullivan KM, Muraro P, Tyndall A. Hematopoietic cell transplantation for autoimmune disease: updates from Europe and the United States. Biol Blood Marrow Transplant 2010;16(1 Suppl):S48–56.
67. Majhail NS, Mau LW, Denzen EM, et al. Costs of autologous and allogeneic hematopoietic cell transplantation in the United States: a study using a large national private claims database. Bone Marrow Transplant 2013;48(2):294–300.
68. Broder MS, Quock TP, Chang E, et al. The cost of hematopoietic stem-cell transplantation in the United States. Am Health Drug Benefits 2017;10(7):366–74.
69. Kopylov U, Afif W. Risk of infections with biological agents. Gastroenterol Clin North Am 2014;43(3):509–24.
70. Tappenden P, Saccardi R, Confavreux C, et al. Autologous haematopoietic stem cell transplantation for secondary progressive multiple sclerosis: an exploratory cost-effectiveness analysis. Bone Marrow Transplant 2010;45(6):1014–21.

71. Sullivan KM, Horwitz M, Osunkwo I, et al. Shared decision-making in hematopoietic stem cell transplantation for sickle cell disease. Biol Blood Marrow Transplant 2018;24(5):883–4.
72. Verburg RJ, Sont JK, Vliet Vlieland TP, et al. High dose chemotherapy followed by autologous peripheral blood stem cell transplantation or conventional pharmacological treatment for refractory rheumatoid arthritis? A Markov decision analysis. J Rheumatol 2001;28(4):719–27.
73. Burt RK, Traynor A, Statkute L, et al. Nonmyeloablative hematopoietic stem cell transplantation for systemic lupus erythematosus. JAMA 2006;295(5):527–35.

Should Platelet-Rich Plasma or Stem Cell Therapy Be Used to Treat Osteoarthritis?

Hani Rashid, DO[a], C. Kent Kwoh, MD[a,b,*]

KEYWORDS

- Osteoarthritis • Knee osteoarthritis • Stem cells • Platelet-rich plasma
- Regenerative medicine • Meta-analyses • Randomized controlled clinical trials

KEY POINTS

- There are no FDA-approved disease-modifying osteoarthritis drugs (DMOADs) available for knee osteoarthritis, which has led to a growing demand for more effective nonoperative treatment options.
- Although platelet-rich plasma and mesenchymal stem cell therapy have been marketed to treat a variety of disorders, including knee osteoarthritis, none of these therapies have been approved for use in osteoarthritis.
- Platelet-rich plasma and mesenchymal stem cell therapy offer the potential to modify the natural course of knee osteoarthritis using cell-based technology.
- Much of the evidence to support the use of either intra-articular platelet-rich plasma or mesenchymal stem cell therapy is of low quality, heterogenous, and at a high risk of bias.
- There is a large degree of heterogeneity, in terms of study designs and measured outcomes, among the published data investigating the use of platelet-rich plasma or mesenchymal stem cell therapy to treat knee osteoarthritis.

PREVALENCE AND IMPACT OF OSTEOARTHRITIS

Osteoarthritis (OA) is the most common musculoskeletal disorder, an enormously costly societal burden, and the leading cause of functional decline, mobility limitations, and disability in the aging population.[1] OA has been designated as a serious disease by the Food and Drug Administration (FDA) for the reasons summarized in **Box 1**.[2,3]

Disclosure Statement: H. Rashid has no relevant financial disclosures to report. C.K. Kwoh has consulting relationships with Astellas, GSK, Fidia, Thusane, Taiwan Liposome Corporation, Regulus, Regeneron, EMD Serono, and Express Scripts.
[a] Division of Rheumatology, University of Arizona College of Medicine, 1501 North Campbell Avenue, PO Box 245093, Tucson, AZ 85724, USA; [b] University of Arizona Arthritis Center, University of Arizona College of Medicine, 1501 North Campbell Avenue, PO Box 245093, Tucson, AZ 85724, USA
* Corresponding author. 1501 North Campbell Avenue, PO Box 245093, Tucson, AZ 85724.
E-mail address: ckwoh@arthritis.arizona.edu

Rheum Dis Clin N Am 45 (2019) 417–438
https://doi.org/10.1016/j.rdc.2019.04.010
rheumatic.theclinics.com

Box 1
Osteoarthritis is a serious disease

Highly prevalent globally
- 240 million people

Prevalence and risk factors are increasing
- Third most rapidly rising condition

No known cure
- No approved treatments to stop the progression of OA

Significant impact in years of life lost because of disability
- 2.4% of all years of life lost because of disability; 10% severe disability

Significant impact on and by comorbid conditions
- Obesity, diabetes, depression, cardiovascular disease, nonalcoholic steatohepatitis

Increased risk of dying prematurely
- 10%–20% relative increase in mortality

Loss of productivity; early retirement; loss of retirement savings
- Greater than 1% Gross Domestic Product in United States

High economic burden to individuals and society
- Total joint replacement numbers rising globally

Natural history of disease progression with no known remission
- ~30% need total joint replacement over 10 years

No proven interventions yet available to stop the progression
- Weight loss and exercise as preventative measures

Current therapies have small treatment effect, are costly, and associated with life-threatening adverse effects
- Nonsteroidal anti-inflammatory drug deaths, opioid crisis

Data from Global Burden of Disease Study C. Global, regional, and national incidence, prevalence, and years lived with disability for 301 acute and chronic diseases and injuries in 188 countries, 1990-2013: a systematic analysis for the Global Burden of Disease Study 2013. Lancet (London, England). 2015;386(9995):743–800. Epub 06/07. https://doi.org/10.1016/S0140-6736(1560692-4). PubMed PMID: 26063472 and OARSI. Osteoarthritis: a serious disease, Submitted to the U.S. Food and Drug Administration https://www.oarsi.org/sites/default/files/library/2018/pdf/oarsi_white_paper_oa_serious_disease121416_1.pdf [March 19, 2019].

Despite its prevalence and enormous impact on public health, OA remains poorly understood. There are currently no FDA-approved disease-modifying OA drugs (DMOADs) to prevent, slow, or halt OA structural changes despite an abundance of potential candidates and clinical trials. Damage evolves over decades with a variable preclinical course, challenging efforts to target and test potential therapeutic strategies.[1] The only effective treatment of end-stage OA is joint replacement.

DEFINITION AND CLINICAL FEATURES

OA is a disease of synovial joints that encompasses the pathophysiologic changes that result from alterations in joint structure caused by failed repair of joint damage and the individual's illness experience, which is most characteristically manifested by pain. The natural history of OA is depicted schematically in **Fig. 1**. One or more triggering events initiate the disease process in a susceptible individual. Aging-related cellular and tissue changes that may occur either before or after the triggering events may increase susceptibility. Currently, clinically detectable OA is defined by the

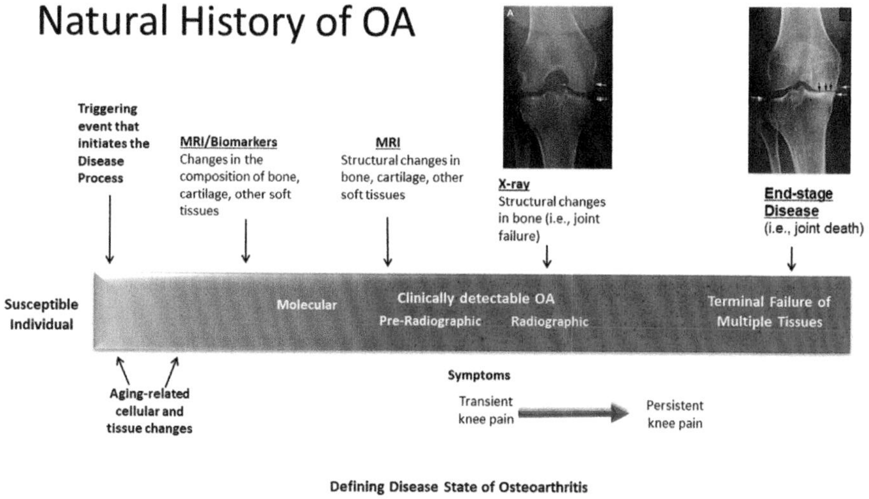

Fig. 1. The natural history of OA.

presence of abnormalities on plain radiographs. Unfortunately, this stage occurs late in the disease course and is indicative of "joint failure." Depending on the joint and other circumstances, symptoms may precede or follow evidence of clinically detectable radiographic OA. Because there are no DMOADs that slow disease progression, patients may progress to end-stage disease (ie, joint death), where the only effective treatment is joint replacement.[4] Several DMOADs have failed in clinical trials, in part because radiographs are an insensitive and nonspecific measure of OA onset and progression. The current research challenge is to identify preradiographic OA through morphologic changes in joint structures that are detectable by MRI or at an even earlier stage of preclinical OA before the onset of symptoms, when molecular changes in joint structures are detectable by compositional MRI or other biomarkers.

The main clinical feature of OA is pain, but radiographic features of OA may be evident before the characteristic pain pattern of OA is present. Pain is generally worse with activity and/or weight-bearing and better with rest. Early in the disease course, pain tends to be transient. With disease progression, pain tends to be more persistent, and in later stages pain may also occur at rest.[5] The cause of the pain associated with OA is unclear and is likely to be heterogeneous. Pain may be the result of an interaction among structural pathology; the motor, sensory, and autonomic innervation of the joint and pain processing at the spinal and cortical levels; and specific individual and environmental factors.[6] There may be peripheral sensitization as a result of hyperalgesia and central sensitization that leads to pain persistence. Allodynia may also be present. In addition, there are several patient-specific factors that may modify pain reception and pain reporting. Patients' affective status, such as depression, anxiety, and anger, may all impact the level of pain reported. Similarly, their cognitive status, including pain beliefs, expectations, memories of past pain experiences, and communication skills all may determine how pain is reported. Studies have shown that demographic factors, such as age, sex, socioeconomic status, race, ethnicity, and cultural background, may also impact pain reporting.[6] Sources of pain in OA include bone marrow lesions in subchondral bone; periostitis with osteophyte formation; subchondral microfractures; and bone ischemia caused by decreased blood flow and/or elevated interosseous pressure, inflammation in the synovium, and irritation of nerve endings by osteophytes.[7]

OSTEOARTHRITIS PATHOGENESIS AND PATHOLOGY

Osteoarthritis Pathogenesis

Although OA was once considered a disease caused by cartilage wear and tear, it is now known to be a complex condition that affects the whole joint, including accumulated changes to bone, synovium, and soft tissue, such as menisci.[8,9] Cartilage, subchondral bone, and synovium likely all play key roles in the pathogenesis of OA. Cartilage architecture and biochemistry are regulated by chondrocytes in response to chemical and mechanical changes. Activated chondrocytes produce inflammatory cytokines (eg, interleukin [IL]-1β, tumor necrosis factor-α) and matrix-degrading enzymes (eg, metalloproteinases, a disintegrin and metalloproteinase with thrombospondin-like motifs [ADAMTS]). The innate immune system is also activated in OA. Chrondrocytes express toll-like receptors, and complement expression and activation are high in osteoarthritic joints. The structure and composition of the cortical plate and trabecular bone are abnormal in OA. Endochondral ossification is reinitiated in OA, accompanied by the formation of osteophytes and subchondral cysts. Osteoblasts, in response to mechanical stimulation, may produce inflammatory cytokines and degradative enzymes, also affecting the cartilage. Subchondral bone remodeling may also result from increased loading through loss of cartilage integrity. Synovitis is common in early OA and persists through later stages. Production of joint lubricants (ie, hyaluronic acid [HA], lubricin) by synoviocytes is suboptimal in OA. Like chondrocytes and osteoblasts, synoviocytes also produce inflammatory mediators and degradative enzymes. Synovitis is associated with symptomatic OA development and progression.

The pathology of OA is seen in **Fig. 2**. OA commonly involves the entire joint. Cartilage degradation results in fibrillation, thinning, and, ultimately, loss of cartilage down to subchondral bone, leaving areas of denuded bone. Pathologic changes include: changes in subchondral bone with thickening, development of bone marrow lesions (which leads to subchondral bone cysts), formation of marginal osteophytes, and bone remodeling with bone attrition that produces changes in bone curvature. There is often weakness of the bridging periarticular muscles. If present, the menisci degenerate and may extrude beyond the bony margins. It is difficult to say which of these processes occurs first, but in later stages, all of these features may be present. Changes in the synovium in OA include synovial hyperplasia, perivascular aggregates of small mononuclear cells, subintimal fibrosis, and increased vascularity.[10]

The characteristic radiographic features of OA are the result of pathologic changes. Joint space narrowing is believed to be a consequence of cartilage loss. Osteophytes may be a consequence of marginal lipping and outgrowths of bone. Subchondral bone cysts and sclerosis may be the result of osteonecrosis and healing of microfractures. Altered bone contours may be caused by bone attrition and remodeling of bone surfaces.

Risk Factors and Osteoarthritis Phenotypes

Several factors can increase the likelihood of developing OA, and these risk factors are divided into systemic- and joint-level risk factors.[1,11] Older age is a well-known risk factor for OA.[12] Women, compared with men, are more likely to develop hand, foot, and knee OA.[13] African-Americans, compared with whites, are more likely to develop symptomatic knee and hip OA.[11] Certain gene variants may predispose individuals to OA development.[14] Obesity and hyperlipidemia are risk factors for the development of knee, hip, and hand OA.[13] High bone mineral density can increase the risk of developing lower extremity OA.[15,16] Particular bone/joint shapes (eg, pistol grip deformity

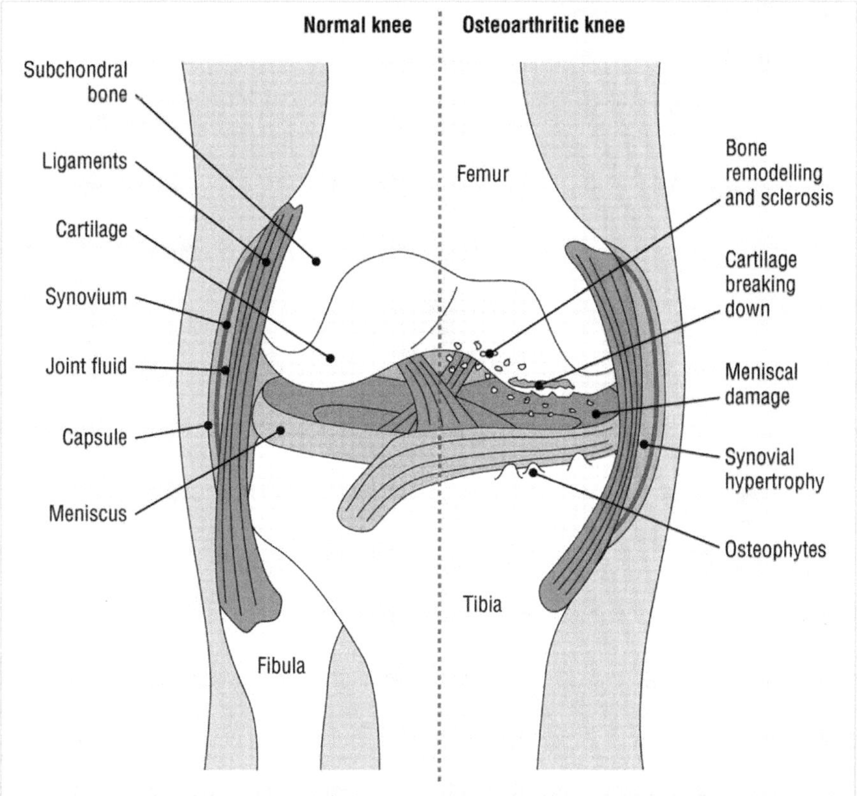

Fig. 2. Pathology of OA. Schematic of the knee joint depicting the synovial joint tissues affected in OA. Consistent with the theory that OA is a disease of the whole synovial joint. (*Data form* Hunter DJ, Felson DT. Osteoarthritis. BMJ (Clinical research ed). 2006;332(7542):639–42. Epub 2006/03/18. https://doi.org/10.1136/bmj.332.7542.639. PubMed PMID: 16543327; PMCID: PMC1403209 and Hunter DJ. Osteoarthritis. Best practice & research Clinical rheumatology. 2011;25(6):801–14. Epub 2012/01/24. https://doi.org/10.1016/j.berh.2011.11.008. PubMed PMID: 22265262.)

of the hip) may increase the risk of developing hip and knee OA.[17] Knee malalignment is associated with worsening of knee OA. Particular occupations (eg, construction work), sports activities associated with injury, and prior joint surgery can predispose people to early localized OA.[11] Ligamental injury, meniscal tear, and cartilage damage have been associated with subsequent OA development. The diversity of risk factors predisposing an individual to OA suggests that a wide variety of insults to the joints, including biomechanical trauma, chronic articular inflammation, and genetic and metabolic factors, can contribute to or trigger the cascade of events that result in the characteristic pathologic features of OA described previously.

A phenotype is defined as a combination of disease attributes that describes differences between patients as they relate to distinct outcomes of interest.[18] Knee OA is a heterogeneous disease with varying phenotypes. There is growing consensus that these variations result from the existence of different phenotypes that may represent different mechanisms of the disease (**Fig. 3**).[19–22] OA may occur as the result of several different pathways that ultimately degenerate into joint failure, a disease process that effects the total joint, including the subchondral bone, ligaments, joint capsule, synovial

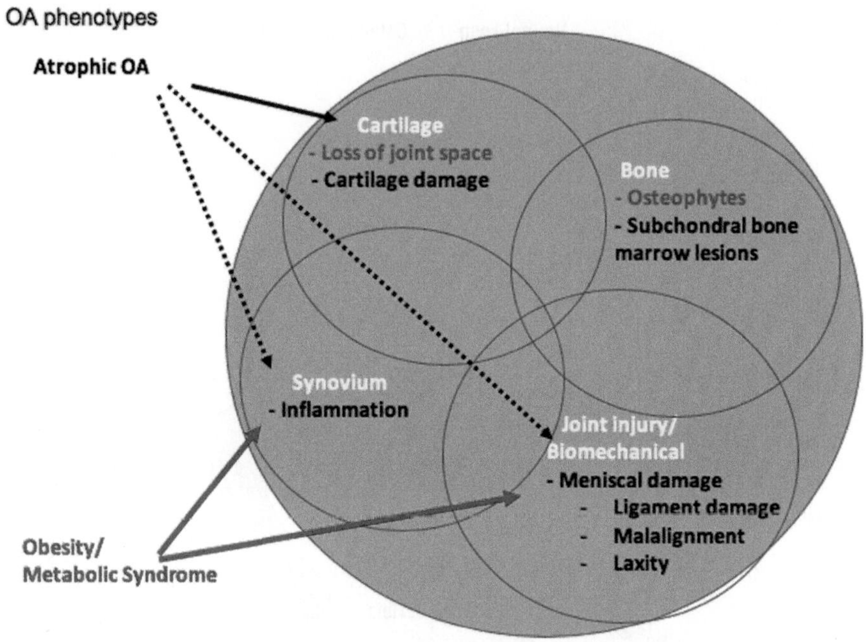

Fig. 3. Knee osteoarthritis phenotypes. A cartilage-centric phenotype is manifested by loss of joint space on radiographs and cartilage damage/loss on MRI. A bone-centric phenotype is expressed by osteophytes on radiographs and subchondral marrow lesions on MRI. A joint injury/biomechanical-centric phenotype is based on joint laxity on physical examination, malalignment on radiographs, and meniscal damage and/or ligament damage on MRI. A synovium-centric phenotype is manifested by joint swelling on physical examination and low-grade inflammation as evidenced by effusion-synovitis and Hoffa-synovitis on MRI.

membrane, periarticular muscles, peripheral nerves, menisci (when present), and articular cartilage.[9] These pathways may consist of abnormal intra-articular and extra-articular processes involving a combination of biomechanical, biochemical, and genetic factors. Examples of these pathways include bone trauma and repetitive injury; malalignment; joint instability caused by muscle weakness and ligamentous laxity; nerve injury, neuronal sensitization, and/or hyperexcitability; low-grade systemic inflammation caused by subacute metabolic syndrome; or local inflammation caused by synovitis. The destruction of the joint, including loss of articular cartilage, is therefore best viewed as the final product of a variety of possible etiologic factors (see **Fig. 3**).

Treatment that targets the mechanism underlying one phenotype may not be effective for a different phenotype. Recognition of different disease phenotypes is crucial so that clinicians may tailor their disease management depending on the specific phenotypes present. Because of the lack of a DMOAD, there has been an increasing number of investigations into the use of platelet-rich plasma (PRP) or stem cell therapy for OA. Because of the large number of studies in the published literature, this review focuses on the use of PRP or stem cell therapy for knee OA because this is the most common type of OA where these interventions are being used.

PLATELET-RICH PLASMA

PRP has become increasingly well known among the public, in large part because of the early adoption of this therapeutic modality by many high-profile international athletes and the presumed safety of this therapeutic approach. Many physicians of various specialties offer PRP injections to their patients in their own outpatient clinics as a cash-based treatment because third-party reimbursement is generally not available for this procedure. Most rheumatologists and orthopedic surgeons have been asked about PRP, either by patients or colleagues seeking effective nonoperative treatment of OA. Published studies are reviewed to provide evidence-based treatment recommendations. There have been several meta-analyses examining the effects of PRP and mesenchymal stem cell (MSC) in patients with knee OA. Measured outcomes typically focus on pain, physical function, radiographic findings, and adverse events.

The use of PRP for knee OA is based on evidence from basic science studies, *in vitro* studies, and animal studies.[23] PRP is derived from autologous plasma, with a concentration of platelets. Because platelets contain a variety of growth factors, coagulation factors, adhesion molecules, cytokines, chemokines, and integrins that are released when activated, the beneficial effects of PRP are thought to be caused by a combination of anabolic growth factors, anti-inflammatory mediators, and several clotting factors, including fibrinogen, which provides a scaffolding effect. This combination is thought to stimulate chondrocyte and MSC proliferation, promote chondrocyte synthesis of aggrecan and collagen type II, drive MSC chondrogenic differentiation, prevent chondrocyte and MSC apoptosis, and diminish the catabolic effects of inflammatory cytokines (**Figs. 4–5**).[23]

There is substantial variability in the preparation of PRP, however, and potential sources of variability are summarized in **Tables 1** and **2**, and **Fig. 6**.

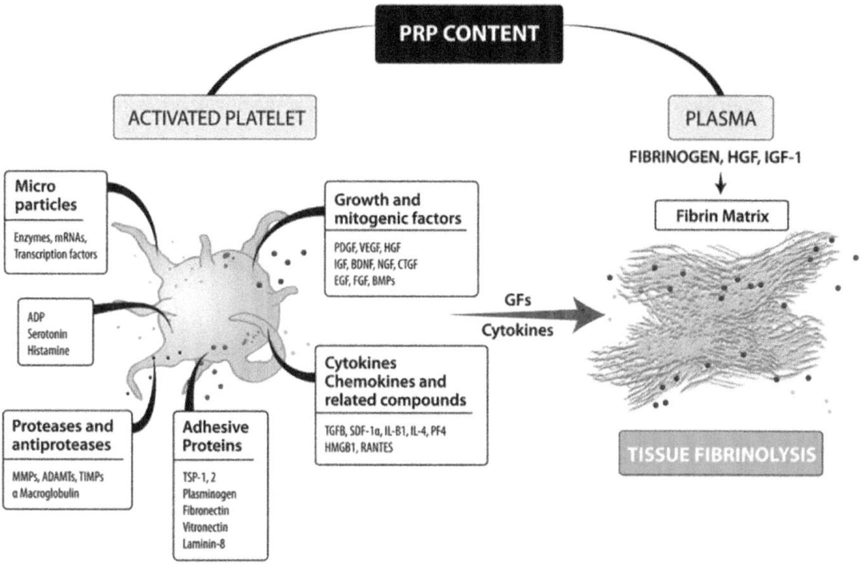

Fig. 4. Illustration of some biologic mediators of PRP that govern tissue repair by still poorly understood mechanisms. (*From* Sánchez M, Garate A, Delgado D, Padilla S. Platelet-rich plasma, an adjuvant biological therapy to assist peripheral nerve repair. Neural regeneration research 2017;12(1):47–52. https://doi.org/10.4103/1673-5374.198973. PubMed PMID: 28250739; with permission; Lane NE, Shidara K, Wise BL. Osteoarthritis year in review 2016: clinical. Osteoarthritis Cartilage. 2017;25(2):209–215.)

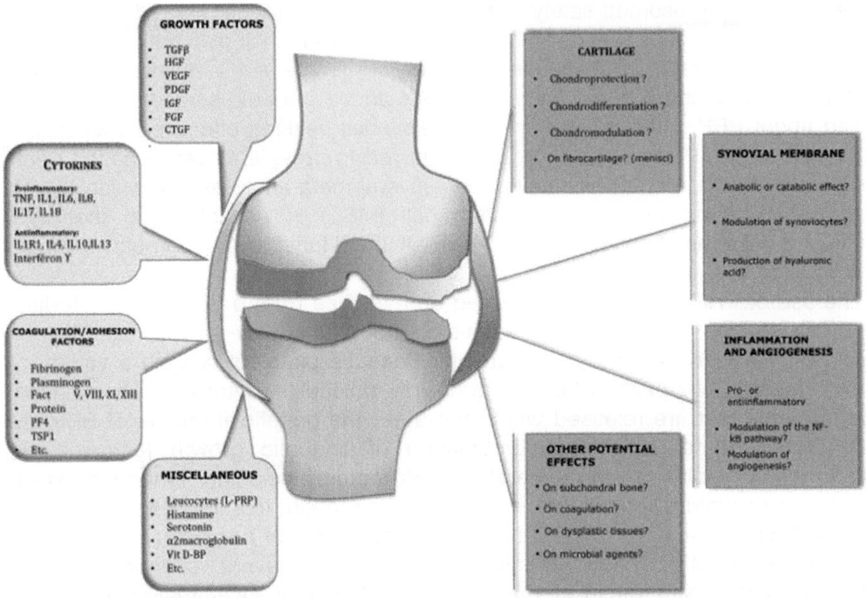

Fig. 5. Main components of PRP, with their potential effects on the osteoarthritis process. (*From* Ornetti P, Nourissat G, Berenbaum F, et al. Does platelet-rich plasma have a role in the treatment of osteoarthritis? Joint Bone Spine. 2016;83(1):31–6. Epub 2015/07/15. https://doi.org/10.1016/j.jbspin.2015.05.002; with permission.)

Meta-analyses of Platelet-Rich Plasma for Knee Osteoarthritis

There have been several meta-analyses or systematic reviews that have attempted to elucidate the efficacy of PRP in the treatment of knee OA.[24–27] Khoshbin and colleagues[24] conducted a systematic review, including six randomized controlled trials

Table 1
Variability in PRP preparation techniques

Collection	Isolation and Concentration	Final Preparation
Initial volume Type and operation of the collecting tube Anticoagulant	PRP system: autologous conditioned plasma, custom systems, or not specified Number of centrifugations: single, double, or not specified Centrifugation revolutions per minute: 1800–3500 rpm Duration of centrifugation: 8–15 min per centrifugation; total duration 8–25 min White blood cell concentration per mL: 0–1.2 × whole blood to 2.3 (10^{7}) or not specified Platelet concentration per mL: >6 (10^7) to >6.8 (10^8) or 5 × whole blood or not specified Complete automation vs human separation	Activating agent: calcium chloride, calcium gluconate, thrombin, batroxobin, not specified or not used Number of PRP injections: 2, 3, or 4 Interval between injections: 1–4 wk Volume of injection: 3–8 mL Location of injection: superolateral, lateral, peripatellar, or not specified

Table 2
Meta-analyses and systemic reviews of PRP

	Khoshbin et al,[24] 2013	Chang et al,[27] 2014	Laudy et al,[25] 2015	Zhang et al,[28] 2018
Date of review	Week 6, 2013	September 2013	June 2014	September 2017
RCTs	4	5	6	10
Prospective nonrandomized	2	3	4	3
Single-arm studies	0	8	0	0
Patients, n	264	1543	1110	1520
Comparator	HA-5 NS-1	HA-6 NS-1	HA-8 NS-1	HA-13 NS-0
Spins, n (if noted)		Single spinning vs double spinning	Single spinning vs double spinning	
WOMAC total score	+	-	+	-
WOMAC pain score, WOMAC physical function score, Lequesne index	-	-	+	-
IKDC score	+	-	-	-
VAS pain score	+	-	+	-
Patient satisfaction	+	-	+	N/A
Adverse events/reactions	+	+	+	N/A
Overall pooled effect size	-	+	-	-

Note: A plus sign indicates formal sensitivity or subgroup analysis was performed, and a minus sign indicates formal sensitivity or subgroup analysis was not performed.

Characteristics of each study included.[26]

Abbreviations: HA, hyaluronic acid; IKDC, International Knee Documentation Committee; N/A, not applicable; NS, normal saline; RCT, randomized controlled trial; VAS, visual analogue scale; WOMAC, Western Ontario and McMaster Universities Osteoarthritis Index.

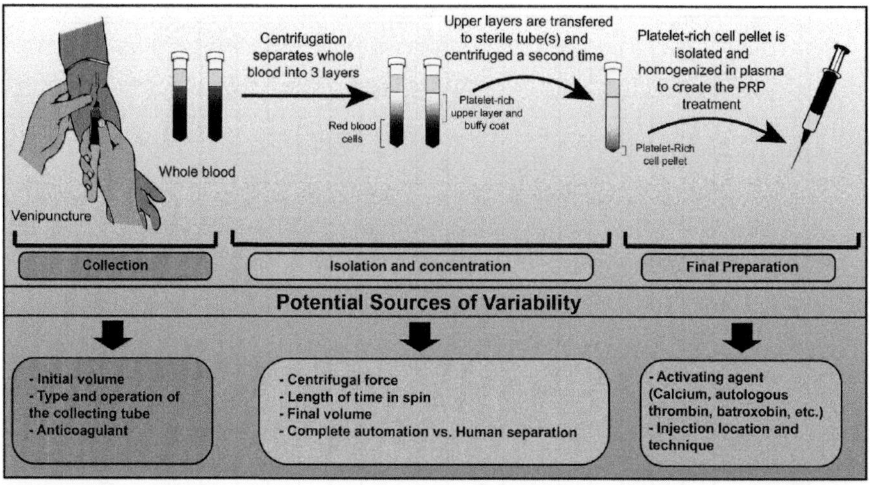

Fig. 6. PRP collection, isolation, and sources of variability. (*From* Jones IA, Togashi RC, Thomas Vangsness C, Jr. The economics and regulation of PRP in the evolving field of orthopedic biologics. Current reviews in musculoskeletal medicine. 2018;11(4):558–65. https://doi.org/10.1007/s12178-018-9514-z. PubMed PMID: 3011699; Dell'Isola A, Allan R, Smith SL, et al. Identification of clinical phenotypes in knee osteoarthritis: a systematic review of the literature. BMC Musculoskelet Disord. 2016;17(1):425.)

(RCTs) and two prospective nonrandomized studies in their final analysis. Functional outcomes were evaluated by Western Ontario and McMaster Universities Osteoarthritis Index (WOMAC) and International Knee Documentation Committee (IKDC) scores, and pain was assessed by Visual Analogue Scale (VAS). At 24 weeks, PRP was favored over control (HA or normal saline) when considering improvement in WOMAC score. IKDC scores were improved in groups receiving PRP over control (HA). There was no statistical difference in VAS scores or patient satisfaction at 24 weeks when comparing groups receiving PRP with control (HA or normal saline). The authors reported that PRP may be effective in the treatment of knee OA.

Chang and colleagues[27] conducted a stratified meta-analysis that included five RCTs, eight open-label prospective studies, and three quasi-experimental studies. One study compared PRP with normal saline, whereas all others used HA as the comparator. Measured outcomes included Knee Injury and Osteoarthritis Outcome Score (KOOS), IKDC, and WOMAC scores. Because of the significant heterogeneity in measured outcomes across studies, pooled effect sizes were estimated from these functional scales and compared across studies. The authors reported that PRP was effective at 12-month follow-up, particularly in those with less cartilage degeneration. They suggested that the effectiveness of PRP was less clear for protocols with less than three injections, use of a single spinning method, and the lack of activation agents.

Laudy and colleagues[25] conducted a systematic review and meta-analysis that included six randomized control and four nonrandomized studies. Pain was assessed by VAS score or WOMAC pain subscale, and function was assessed by the WOMAC physical function subscale, WOMAC total score, or Lequesne index. They found that PRP was more effective than control (placebo or HA) for reducing pain and improving physical function at 6 months postinjection. They reported that PRP may be effective, but there was significant heterogeneity in the study designs (including the type of PRP used and the approach to the spinning of the PRP before use). The level of supporting evidence was also limited because of a high risk of bias.

In 2018, Zhang and colleagues[28] performed a meta-analysis comparing intra-articular PRP with HA in the treatment of knee OA. Ten RCTs and three prospective trials were included in their analysis. Although PRP seemed to improve WOMAC pain scores more effectively than HA (at 6 and 12 months) and VAS pain scores (at 3 and 6 months), the results were not statistically different. The authors concluded that PRP did not seem to be superior to HA in the treatment of knee OA.

Based on their review of three of the previously mentioned analyses,[24,25,27] Campbell and colleagues[26] reported that PRP led to durable and significant improvement in pain and function in patients with knee OA, but emphasized that patients with early degenerative changes seemed to receive the most benefit. Multiple PRP injections seemed to increase the risk of local reactions, however. A major concern with Campbell's findings is that only one RCT from all the RCTs in the three publications that they summarized compared PRP with a single placebo injection,[29] whereas the others most often used HA as the comparator. In the study by Patel and colleagues,[29] it is likely that the investigators and patients were not truly blinded, because those who received PRP received either one or two PRP injections, whereas the normal saline group only underwent one injection. In addition, there was no statistical comparison of the differences in improvement among the three groups.

Randomized Controlled Trials of Platelet-Rich Plasma for Knee Osteoarthritis

Yu and colleagues[30] investigated the use of intra-articular PRP and HA in the treatment of knee OA. Patients were randomized to receive PRP, HA, PRP + HA, or normal saline placebo. Improvement at 12-month follow-up was noted in WOMAC subscales in each of the three treatment arms, but this improvement was compared with each group's respective baseline WOMAC scores rather than with placebo. Whether or not patients receiving saline placebo had similar improvement in the measured indices was not discussed. Despite these shortcomings, the authors reported that levels of tumor necrosis factor-α, IL-1β, and IL-17 decreased in groups receiving HA or PRP and further decreased in the group receiving combination HA and PRP. In contrast, levels of IL-6 increased in groups receiving HA or PRP and further increased in the group receiving combination HA and PRP. The significance of these findings is unclear.

In a superiority designed study Lin and colleagues[31] randomized 87 knees with mild to moderate OA to receive three weekly injections of either PRP, HA, or normal saline placebo. Patients receiving PRP had statistically significant improvement in WOMAC scores compared with placebo at 2, 6, and 12 months, whereas the group receiving HA did not have any improvement compared with placebo, controlling for age, sex, body mass index, and stage of OA. The authors concluded that three intra-articular injections with PRP were superior to three injections of HA or placebo.

Because of the short follow-up periods (ie, between 3 and 12 months), there were no outcome data available on slowing of the progression of radiographic or MRI-detected damage in these studies.

Platelet-Rich Plasma Adverse Events

Most of the meta-analyses and RCTs reviewed thus far describe self-limited pain and swelling after injection of PRP, which were not statistically different from placebo or groups receiving other treatments (ie, HA). Because PRP injections are autologous, systemic transfusion reactions would be unexpected. However, one of the few RCTs comparing PRP with saline placebo reported an increased incidence of local (postinjection pain and stiffness) and systemic (syncope, dizziness, headache, nausea, sweating, and tachycardia) reactions in subjects treated with PRP.[29] Filardo and colleagues[32] reported additional adverse effects with regards to postinjection knee pain and swelling with a double-spinning versus single-spinning PRP preparation.

There are reports of thromboembolic events, such as deep venous thrombosis and pulmonary embolism, occurring in patients receiving PRP following total knee arthroplasty, a surgical procedure known to increase the risk of such events because of postoperative immobilization and other factors.[33] However, we could not find episodes of deep venous thrombosis or pulmonary embolism in patients treated with PRP who did not undergo concomitant total knee arthroplasty.

Cases of viral hepatitis transmission have been reported in patients receiving PRP.[34] The California Department of Public Health attributed a case of hepatitis C virus transmission in one clinic offering PRP to significant infection control breaches including using single-dose medication vials for multiple patients, lack of aseptic technique, and poor hand hygiene.[34] Presumably, the risk of pathogen transmission would approach zero if appropriate precautions are followed because PRP is an autologous treatment.

Platelet-Rich Plasma Conclusion

In clinical trials and nonrandomized studies, PRP is most often compared with HA as a control; rarely is a true control, such as normal saline, used as the comparator. The lack of a true control group in several of the studies included in the previously mentioned meta-analyses group limits the ability to interpret placebo effects because of the use of an invasive treatment. Bannuru and colleagues[35] performed a network meta-analysis of OA studies and found that intra-articular placebos had a higher effect size than oral placebos.

Although many of the studies we reviewed reported that PRP could improve pain and physical function, the evidence to support these assertions was generally of low quality. As described in **Table 1**, there is substantial variability in PRP protocols regarding factors related to isolation, collection, and administration. Furthermore, we noted significant heterogeneity among the study designs and measured outcomes of these meta-analyses. Most of the studies did not follow patients beyond 1 year, raising concerns for long-term durability of treatment, and potential adverse effects on the knee joint, which may not be apparent early in treatment. There is also some suggestion that patients at an earlier stage of cartilage degeneration are more likely to benefit from PRP, but more specifics are needed to be able to define which patients may most benefit from PRP.

STEM CELL THERAPY

Stem cells help to create new cells (and/or recruit cells to damaged locations) in existing healthy tissues and may help repair tissues in areas that are injured or damaged. They have several unique characteristics, including: the ability to self-renew; the ability to divide for a long period of time; and, under certain conditions, the ability to be induced to differentiate into specialized cells with distinct functions. Stem cells are obtained from a variety of sources, including: the inner cell mass of a blastocyst (ie, embryonic stem cells); blood from the umbilical cord of a newborn baby; amniotic fluid; placenta; and from differentiated tissues and organs throughout the body, such as bone marrow and adipose tissue (ie, adult stem cells). Induced pluripotent stem cells can also be derived from the large pool of differentiated cells in the body (eg, skin, fat, muscle). The process of having stem cells differentiate into a specific tissue of interest is complex and not an easy endeavor *in vivo*. In addition, whether a specific tissue source might be optimal for a given clinical situation has not yet been established.[36,37] MSCs have been characterized as an injury drugstore with a pluripotent capacity to differentiate into a variety of mesenchymal tissues (**Fig. 7**).[36] The healing potential of MSCs is based on their immunomodulatory and trophic properties (**Figs. 8–10**).[36]

Meta-analyses of Mesenchymal Stem Cells

Iijima and colleagues[38] recently performed a meta-analysis of seven RCTs and 28 nonrandomized studies to better define the current evidence for the efficacy and safety of MSCs in the treatment of knee OA. They found that treating knee OA with MSCs significantly improved pain as assessed by VAS scores (mean follow-up period of 14.0 $\pm$ 12.9 months, decreased to 12 months if only RCTs included). Physical function, as assessed by the WOMAC subscale, also was significantly improved in patients treated with MSCs (mean follow-up period of 17.0 $\pm$ 10.8 months).

When they limited their analysis to RCTs, however, the gains in pain relief and physical function were attenuated. The authors warned that the conclusions they had drawn from their meta-analysis were based on "low" or "very low" quality evidence based on the GRADE approach,[39] and attributed this to high risk of bias, flawed study designs, heterogeneity, and wide confidence intervals in the studies analyzed. They

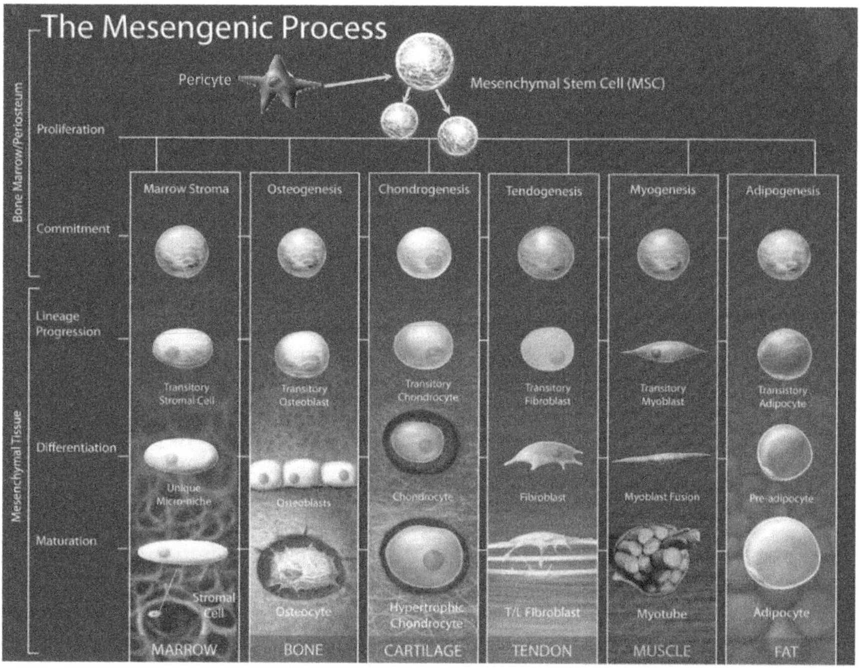

Fig. 7. The mesengenic process. The original version of this figure was generated in the late 1980s (Caplan, 1991, 1994) and has been modernized in this rendition. The figure proposes that an MSC exists in the bone marrow and that its progeny can be induced to enter one of several mesenchymal lineage pathways. The lineage format was constructed from what was known about the hematopoietic lineage pathway, and this figure depicts the predicted differentiation hierarchy of the most prominent candidate lineages. (*From* Caplan AI, Correa D. The MSC: an injury drugstore. Cell Stem Cell. 2011 Jul 8;9(1):11-5. https://doi.org/10.1016/j.stem.2011.06.008; with permission.)

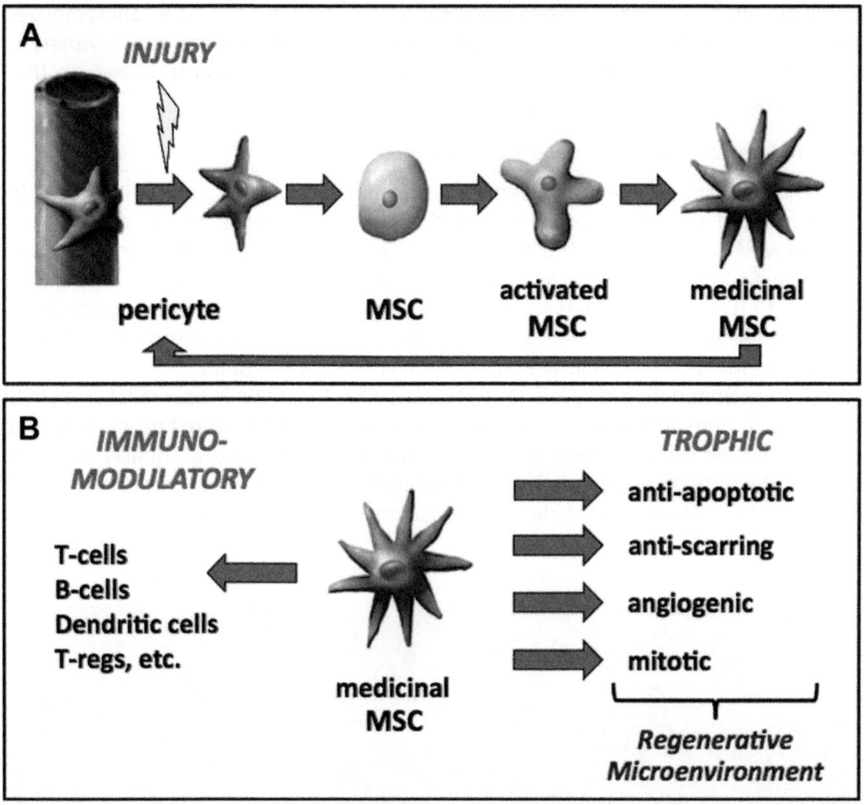

Fig. 8. MSCs are immunomodulatory and trophic. (*A*) The proposed sequential activation of pericytes as a response to injury. Local vessel damage affects resident pericytes and liberates them from functional contact with blood vessels to become activated MSCs. On immune activation, these mobilized, "medicinal" MSCs secrete factors that organize a regenerative microenvironment. Subsequent repair is reinforced when activated MSCs reacquire a stabilizing pericyte phenotype in the abluminal space. (*B*) The bioactive molecules secreted by medicinal MSCs are immunomodulatory and affect a variety of immune cell lineages.[29] Other secreted molecules establish a regenerative microenvironment by establishing a powerful trophic field. (*From* Caplan AI, Correa D. The MSC: an injury drugstore. Cell stem cell. 2011;9(1):11–5. Epub 2011/07/06. https://doi.org/10.1016/j.stem.2011.06.008; with permission.)

drew attention to the fact that many of the studies evaluated in their meta-analysis were authored by the same group of investigators.

Borakati and colleagues[40] performed a meta-analysis that assessed improvement in VAS-measured pain in patients with knee OA. They quantitatively analyzed 13 studies and qualitatively analyzed 36 studies. Unlike some of the meta-analyses that preceded it, this analysis only included studies that used control groups without chondrogenic cellular therapy because elucidating the true efficacy of MSCs requires comparison with a control group that is not receiving another form of regenerative therapy.

Borakati and colleagues[40] found a reduction in pain (preferentially measured by VAS) in patients treated with MSCs, using the value closest to 1-year follow-up to provide consistency. They called attention to significant limitations in the studies

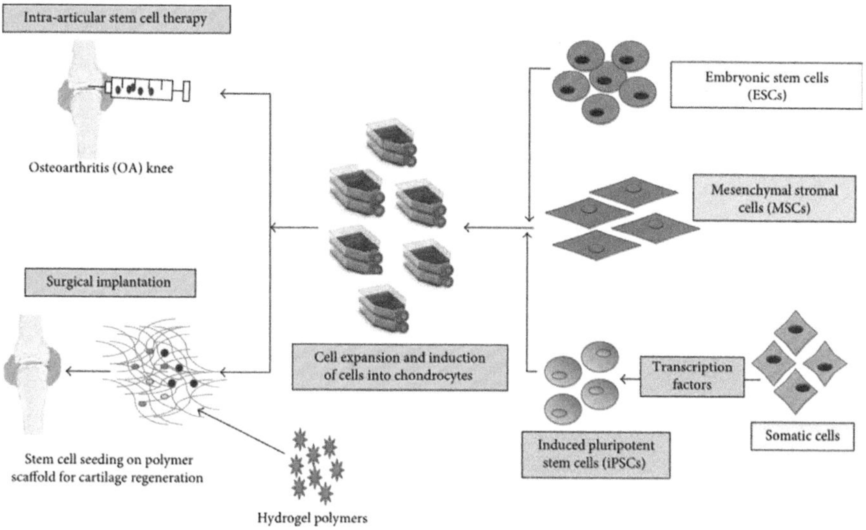

Fig. 9. Schematic of stem cell–based therapy in OA. (*From* Dubey NK, Mishra VK, Dubey R, Syed-Abdul S, Wang JR, Wang PD, Deng W-P. Combating osteoarthritis through stem cell therapies by rejuvenating cartilage: a review. Stem cells international. 2018;2018:5421019. https://doi.org/10.1155/2018/5421019; with permission; Yu W, Xu P, Huang G, et al. Clinical therapy of hyaluronic acid combined with platelet-rich plasma for the treatment of knee osteoarthritis. Exp Ther Med. 2018;16(3):2119–2125.)

reviewed, notably the observational nature of most of the analyzed studies and the generally poor quality of the studies (attributed to a lack of randomization and blinding). In addition, there was significant heterogeneity across the studies analyzed, in study design and outcomes measured. There was also variation in the method of placing the MSCs (injection vs transplantation), the quantity of stem cells injected, the contents of the injectate (HA, PRP), and the coincident surgical procedures (microfractures, arthroscopic debridement, or high tibial osteotomy).

Yubo and colleagues[41] performed a meta-analysis to evaluate the therapeutic efficacy and safety of MSCs in the treatment of knee OA. Eleven studies were included in the final analysis. The authors found that MSC therapy brought improvement in pain as measured by VAS score (at 6, 12, and 24 months) and physical function as measured by IKDC (at 24 months). WOMAC scores also improved at 12-month follow-up. They did not find an increase in adverse events.

Recent Randomized Controlled Trials of Mesenchymal Stem Cells

Several additional RCTs have been reported since the previously mentioned meta-analyses were published. Although some have continued to simply test the efficacy of MSCs, others have delved into more complex protocols, such as assessing differing MSC doses and using combination with PRP.

Emadedin and colleagues[42] published findings from their single-center, randomized, triple-blind (subjects, investigators, and data analysts all blinded), placebo-controlled phase 1/2 trial evaluating implantation of MSCs versus normal saline in a group of 43 patients. MSCs were derived from bone marrow aspiration in all patients, although only patients in the treatment arm received intra-articular MSC injection. MSCs were found to improve WOMAC pain, WOMAC function, and painless walking distance compared with placebo at 6-month follow-up.

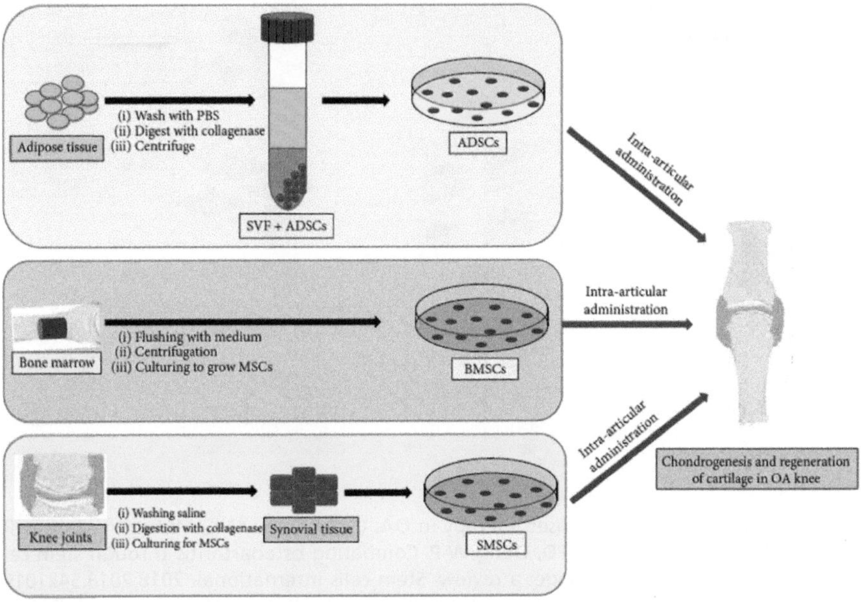

Fig. 10. An overview of isolation procedure of various stem cells and their administration in the OA knee joint. ADSCs, adipose-derived stem cells; BMSCs, bone marrow–derived stem cells; PBS, phosphate-buffered saline; SVF, stromal vascular fraction. (*From* Dubey NK, Mishra VK, Dubey R, Syed-Abdul S, Wang JR, Wang PD, Deng W-P. Combating osteoarthritis through stem cell therapies by rejuvenating cartilage: a review. Stem cells international. 2018;2018:5421019. https://doi.org/10.1155/2018/5421019; with permission; Yu W, Xu P, Huang G, et al. Clinical therapy of hyaluronic acid combined with platelet-rich plasma for the treatment of knee osteoarthritis. Exp Ther Med. 2018;16(3):2119–2125.)

Shapiro and colleagues[43] performed an elegant study in which patients with bilateral knee OA essentially served as their own control subjects: each of the 25 patients in the study received an intra-articular injection of bone marrow aspirate concentrate in one knee and saline in the contralateral knee. Pain was assessed by OARSI Intermittent and Constant Osteoarthritis Pain and VAS scores. Patients reported similar improvements in pain in both knees at 1 week, 3 months, and 6 months postintervention.

Bastos and colleagues[44] randomized 18 patients to receive either intra-articular injection of MSCs or MSCs plus PRP. KOOS subscales were the primary outcomes measured at 12-month follow-up. They reported improvement in most KOOS subscales in the MSC and MSC plus PRP treated groups, suggesting that PRP added no clinical benefit when added to an MSC injectate in the treatment of knee OA.

Mesenchymal Stem Cells Adverse Events

Because OA is associated with significant morbidity, but with a limited effect on mortality, consideration of the safety of treatments, such as stem cell therapy, is a critical consideration in medical decision making.[45] Although use of MSCs seems to be safe based on the published literature available, serious adverse effects including death, infection, pulmonary embolism, and tumors have been reported with the use of MSCs for a variety of diseases.[46] The most frequently reported adverse events reported have been postinjection joint pain and joint swelling, which was self-limited in most cases. There has been at least one report of post-treatment articular fibrosis in a patient being treated for knee OA with MSC implantation.[47]

Other potential safety concerns for unproven stem cell treatments include: administration site reactions, the ability of cells to move from placement sites and change into inappropriate cell types or multiply, failure of cells to work as expected, and the growth of tumors.[48]

Marketing of Platelet-Rich Plasma and Mesenchymal Stem Cells

PRP and MSC therapy are being increasingly marketed directly to consumers, often eluding the reach of regulatory bodies.[49,50] Many patients desperate for curing a variety of ailments ranging from alopecia to OA flock to purported clinics in the hopes of finding a miracle treatment. These clinics are not particularly hard to find; Turner and Knoepfler[51] found that 351 businesses in the United States engage in direct-to-consumer marketing of stem cell treatments at a total of 570 clinics nationwide.

According to one review by Piuzzi and colleagues,[52] the mean price for treating one OA knee with stem cell therapy was $5156, nearly 10% of the median annual American income. Although the same group also reported that the mean price of a single intra-articular knee injection with PRP was $714, one should consider that PRP is often given in a series of injections.[53] Certainly, there is only a select group of patients that can afford such an expense, although one can imagine that most patients who are investigating PRP and MSC therapy may have already spent a considerable amount of their savings on more well-established treatments.

Physicians have a responsibility to inform such patients that by diverting their financial resources to these therapies, they may be foregoing effective treatments that may be the standard of care to treat their disease.[50] To that end, California now requires its more than 100 stem cell clinics to disclose that their treatments are not approved by the FDA and tell their patients that they should consult with their physicians before proceeding with the therapy.[54] The FDA has put out an advisory for consumers warning them about the unproven efficacy of stem cell therapies and their potential for adverse effects, as seen in **Box 2**.[48] PRP currently only has FDA clearance for its use to enhance bone graft handling properties in orthopedic procedures.[55] However, the FDA has not issued advisory statements to patients seeking off-label use of PRP, such as for OA.

Although most physicians have some inkling that the cost of the cash-only business of stem cell therapy is substantial, they may not know that some patients, including at least one infant receiving treatment, have died following treatment.[56] In addition, many patients have been deceived by individuals falsely portraying themselves as physicians into paying large sums of money for stem cell therapies to treat incurable diseases, such as amyotrophic lateral sclerosis, multiple sclerosis, and Parkinson disease.[57]

There was a time where patients received much of their medical information directly from health professionals; this time has come and gone. Physicians are all too aware that most patients now thoroughly research treatment options for their conditions online before their first consultation with a physician, often through social media outlets rather than reputable medical Web sites. Although physicians would agree that patients should be knowledgeable about their diseases, the sources of their knowledge should be scrutinized.

Ramkumar and colleagues[58] investigated social media content across a variety of platforms, including Facebook, Instagram, LinkedIn, and Twitter. They found that most stem cell information available on social media was in the form of advertisements that primarily touted potential benefits without including the necessary disclosures of risks and limitations of treatment. A paltry 8% of the social media content pertained to patient-reported experiences with stem cell therapy. Although their finding that social

Box 2
Advice for people considering stem cell therapies

Stem cell products have the potential to treat many medical conditions and diseases. But for almost all of these products, it is not yet known whether the product has any benefit, or if the product is safe to use.

If you are considering treatment in the United States:

- *Ask if the FDA has reviewed the treatment.* Ask your health care provider to confirm this information. You also can ask the clinical investigator to give you the FDA-issued Investigational New Drug Application number and the chance to review the FDA communication acknowledging the IND. Ask for this information *before* getting treatment–even if the stem cells are your own.
- *Request the facts and ask questions if you do not understand.* To participate in a clinical trial that requires an IND application, you must sign a consent form that explains the experimental procedure. The consent form also identifies the Institutional Review Board (IRB) that assures the protection of the rights and welfare of human subjects. Make sure you understand the entire process and known risks before you sign. You also can ask the study sponsor for the clinical investigator's brochure, which includes a short description of the product and information about its safety and effectiveness.

If you are considering treatment in another country:

- *Learn about regulations that cover products in that country.*
- *Know that the FDA does not have oversight of treatments done in other countries.* The FDA typically has little information about foreign establishments or their stem cell products.
- *Be cautious.* If you are considering a stem cell-based product in a country that may not require regulatory review of clinical studies, it may be hard to know if the experimental treatment is reasonably safe.

From US Food and Drug Administration. FDA Warns about stem cell therapies. Available at https://www.fda.gov/forconsumers/consumerupdates/ucm286155.htm

media may be serving business interests rather than providing useful information to consumers comes as no surprise, it is disheartening to consider that patients may be receiving the bulk of their medical knowledge from industry-supported advertisements.

Mesenchymal Stem Cells Conclusion

There has been an exponential rise in the amount of published data pertaining to the use of MSC therapy in the treatment of knee OA over the past decade. The results of the meta-analyses presented have limitations because of heterogeneity in study design and outcome measures, and high risk of bias. Furthermore, much of the published improvement in pain and function was attenuated when only RCTs were included in the meta-analyses.

Although heterogeneity is to be expected with the study of a new therapeutic modality, guidelines for treatment protocols and study designs for investigating the risk and benefits of MSC therapy are needed. No single version of MSC therapy has been proven to be more effective than others. Given the modest effects noted in the published literature, there needs to be a movement from refinement of techniques to proof of efficacy so that the value derived from MSC treatment is optimized.

We must acknowledge that patients can and will embark on their own journey for "treatment and cures" regardless of effect sizes, *P* values, and confidence intervals. Just as important as the question of MSC efficacy is whether or not the public will seek out MSC therapy. Will patients pay to have painful bone-marrow aspiration, intra-articular injection, or operative intra-articular implantation (with the perioperative risk this entails) of MSCs, to improve their VAS pain score by 1 point for 6 months? Will they accept that most of the studies on MSCs do not demonstrate long-term durability in pain-relief or physical function?

Rather than merely halting disease, MSCs offers the potential to rewrite the natural history of knee OA. In reality, the line between the paradigm of prevention and the paradigm of treatment is blurred when discussing regenerative medical treatment, such as the use of MSCs in the treatment of knee OA. Although injecting or implanting MSCs may regenerate cartilage, and possibly engage in rehabilitation programs to prevent recurrence of degenerative arthritis, confidence in the efficacy and safety of such treatments is currently beyond the reach of rheumatologists, orthopedic surgeons, and other physicians.

SUMMARY

There has been an exponential rise in the amount of published data pertaining to the use of PRP and MSCs in the treatment of knee OA over the past decade. Currently, PRP and MSC therapy seem to offer patients small gains in pain relief and physical function. The quality of the supporting data is suspect, because of considerable heterogeneity among treatment protocols, PRP formulations, MSC formulations, study designs, measured outcomes, lack of comparison with true placebo, and outcome measurements rarely exceeding 12 months. Physicians should maintain a healthy degree of skepticism when discussing these treatment options with patients.

The burgeoning fields of intra-articular PRP and MSC therapy have garnered significant attention from patients, the press, and the medical community. Unfortunately, patients' thirst for knowledge has been frequently quenched by industry-supported advertisements and largely unsubstantiated claims made by unregulated clinics. Despite the lack of robust data supporting the use of either PRP or MSC therapy in the treatment of knee OA, PRP and MSC industries continue to thrive in the absence of true DMOADs to prevent disease onset or progression.

REFERENCES

1. Vina ER, Kwoh CK. Epidemiology of osteoarthritis: literature update. Curr Opin Rheumatol 2018;30(2):160–7.
2. Global Burden of Disease Study 2013 Collaborators. Global, regional, and national incidence, prevalence, and years lived with disability for 301 acute and chronic diseases and injuries in 188 countries, 1990-2013: a systematic analysis for the Global Burden of Disease Study 2013. Lancet 2015;386(9995):743–800.
3. OARSI. Osteoarthritis: a serious disease, Submitted to the U.S. Food and Drug Administration. Available at: https://www.oarsi.org/sites/default/files/library/2018/pdf/oarsi_white_paper_oa_serious_disease121416_1.pdf. Accessed March 19, 2019.
4. Kwoh C. The epidemiology of aging. Epidemiology of osteoarthritis. 1st edition. New York: Springer; 2012. p. 523–36.
5. Hawker GA, Davis AM, French MR, et al. Development and preliminary psychometric testing of a new OA pain measure: an OARSI/OMERACT initiative. Osteoarthritis Cartilage 2008;16(4):409–14.
6. Marchand S. The physiology of pain mechanisms: from the periphery to the brain. Rheum Dis Clin North Am 2008;34(2):285–309.

7. Fitzcharles MA, Shir Y. New concepts in rheumatic pain. Rheum Dis Clin North Am 2008;34(2):267–83.
8. Glyn-Jones S, Palmer AJ, Agricola R, et al. Osteoarthritis. Lancet 2015; 386(9991):376–87.
9. Lane NE, Brandt K, Hawker G, et al. OARSI-FDA initiative: defining the disease state of osteoarthritis. Osteoarthritis Cartilage 2011;19(5):478–82.
10. Scanzello CR, Plaas A, Crow MK. Innate immune system activation in osteoarthritis: is osteoarthritis a chronic wound? Curr Opin Rheumatol 2008;20(5): 565–72.
11. Silverwood V, Blagojevic-Bucknall M, Jinks C, et al. Current evidence on risk factors for knee osteoarthritis in older adults: a systematic review and meta-analysis. Osteoarthritis Cartilage 2015;23(4):507–15.
12. Loeser RF. Age-related changes in the musculoskeletal system and the development of osteoarthritis. Clin Geriatr Med 2010;26(3):371–86.
13. Hunter DJ. Osteoarthritis. Best Pract Res Clin Rheumatol 2011;25(6):801–14.
14. Warner SC, Valdes AM. Genetic association studies in osteoarthritis: is it fairytale? Curr Opin Rheumatol 2017;29(1):103–9.
15. Teichtahl AJ, Wang Y, Wluka AE, et al. Associations between systemic bone mineral density and early knee cartilage changes in middle-aged adults without clinical knee disease: a prospective cohort study. Arthritis Res Ther 2017;19(1):98.
16. Edwards MH, Paccou J, Ward KA, et al. The relationship of bone properties using high resolution peripheral quantitative computed tomography to radiographic components of hip osteoarthritis. Osteoarthritis Cartilage 2017;25(9):1478–83.
17. Saberi Hosnijeh F, Zuiderwijk ME, Versteeg M, et al. Cam deformity and acetabular dysplasia as risk factors for hip osteoarthritis. Arthritis Rheumatol 2017;69(1): 86–93.
18. Pinto LM, Alghamdi M, Benedetti A, et al. Derivation and validation of clinical phenotypes for COPD: a systematic review. Respir Res 2015;16:50.
19. Lane NE, Shidara K, Wise BL. Osteoarthritis year in review 2016: clinical. Osteoarthritis Cartilage 2017;25(2):209–15.
20. Bierma-Zeinstra SM, Verhagen AP. Osteoarthritis subpopulations and implications for clinical trial design. Arthritis Res Ther 2011;13(2):213.
21. Dell'Isola A, Allan R, Smith SL, et al. Identification of clinical phenotypes in knee osteoarthritis: a systematic review of the literature. BMC Musculoskelet Disord 2016;17(1):425.
22. Deveza LA, Melo L, Yamato TP, et al. Knee osteoarthritis phenotypes and their relevance for outcomes: a systematic review. Osteoarthritis Cartilage 2017; 25(12):1926–41.
23. Xie X, Zhang C, Tuan RS. Biology of platelet-rich plasma and its clinical application in cartilage repair. Arthritis Res Ther 2014;16(1):204.
24. Khoshbin A, Leroux T, Wasserstein D, et al. The efficacy of platelet-rich plasma in the treatment of symptomatic knee osteoarthritis: a systematic review with quantitative synthesis. Arthroscopy 2013;29(12):2037–48.
25. Laudy AB, Bakker EW, Rekers M, et al. Efficacy of platelet-rich plasma injections in osteoarthritis of the knee: a systematic review and meta-analysis. Br J Sports Med 2015;49(10):657–72.
26. Campbell KA, Saltzman BM, Mascarenhas R, et al. Does intra-articular platelet-rich plasma injection provide clinically superior outcomes compared with other therapies in the treatment of knee osteoarthritis? A systematic review of overlapping meta-analyses. Arthroscopy 2015;31(11):2213–21.

27. Chang KV, Hung CY, Aliwarga F, et al. Comparative effectiveness of platelet-rich plasma injections for treating knee joint cartilage degenerative pathology: a systematic review and meta-analysis. Arch Phys Med Rehabil 2014;95(3):562–75.
28. Zhang HF, Wang CG, Li H, et al. Intra-articular platelet-rich plasma versus hyaluronic acid in the treatment of knee osteoarthritis: a meta-analysis. Drug Des Devel Ther 2018;12:445–53.
29. Patel S, Dhillon MS, Aggarwal S, et al. Treatment with platelet-rich plasma is more effective than placebo for knee osteoarthritis: a prospective, double-blind, randomized trial. Am J Sports Med 2013;41(2):356–64.
30. Yu W, Xu P, Huang G, et al. Clinical therapy of hyaluronic acid combined with platelet-rich plasma for the treatment of knee osteoarthritis. Exp Ther Med 2018;16(3):2119–25.
31. Lin KY, Yang CC, Hsu CJ, et al. Intra-articular injection of platelet-rich plasma is superior to hyaluronic acid or saline solution in the treatment of mild to moderate knee osteoarthritis: a randomized, double-blind, triple-parallel, placebo-controlled clinical trial. Arthroscopy 2019;35(1):106–17.
32. Filardo G, Kon E, Pereira Ruiz MT, et al. Platelet-rich plasma intra-articular injections for cartilage degeneration and osteoarthritis: single- versus double-spinning approach. Knee Surg Sports Traumatol Arthrosc 2012;20(10):2082–91.
33. Ma N, Wang H, Xu X, et al. Autologous-cell-derived, tissue-engineered cartilage for repairing articular cartilage lesions in the knee: study protocol for a randomized controlled trial. Trials 2017;18(1):519.
34. Foster MA, Grigg C, Hagon J, et al. Notes from the Field. Investigation of hepatitis C virus transmission associated with injection therapy for chronic pain—California, 2015. Morb Mortal Wkly Rep 2016;65:547–9.
35. Bannuru RR, McAlindon TE, Sullivan MC, et al. Effectiveness and implications of alternative placebo treatments: a systematic review and network meta-analysis of osteoarthritis trials. Ann Intern Med 2015;163(5):365–72.
36. Caplan AI, Correa D. The MSC: an injury drugstore. Cell Stem Cell 2011; 9(1):11–5.
37. Aggarwal S, Pittenger MF. Human mesenchymal stem cells modulate allogeneic immune cell responses. Blood 2005;105(4):1815–22.
38. Iijima H, Isho T, Kuroki H, et al. Effectiveness of mesenchymal stem cells for treating patients with knee osteoarthritis: a meta-analysis toward the establishment of effective regenerative rehabilitation. NPJ Regen Med 2018;3(1). https://doi.org/10.1038/s41536-018-0041-8.
39. Balshem H, Helfand M, Schunemann HJ, et al. GRADE guidelines: 3. Rating the quality of evidence. J Clin Epidemiol 2011;64(4):401–6.
40. Borakati A, Mafi R, Mafi P, et al. A systematic review and meta-analysis of clinical trials of mesenchymal stem cell therapy for cartilage repair. Curr Stem Cell Res Ther 2018;13(3):215–25.
41. Yubo M, Yanyan L, Li L, et al. Clinical efficacy and safety of mesenchymal stem cell transplantation for osteoarthritis treatment: a meta-analysis. PLoS One 2017; 12(4):e0175449.
42. Emadedin M, Labibzadeh N, Liastani MG, et al. Intra-articular implantation of autologous bone marrow-derived mesenchymal stromal cells to treat knee osteoarthritis: a randomized, triple-blind, placebo-controlled phase 1/2 clinical trial. Cytotherapy 2018;20(10):1238–46.
43. Shapiro SA, Kazmerchak SE, Heckman MG, et al. A prospective, single-blind, placebo-controlled trial of bone marrow aspirate concentrate for knee osteoarthritis. Am J Sports Med 2017;45(1):82–90.

44. Bastos R, Mathias M, Andrade R, et al. Intra-articular injections of expanded mesenchymal stem cells with and without addition of platelet-rich plasma are safe and effective for knee osteoarthritis. Knee Surg Sports Traumatol Arthrosc 2018;26(11):3342–50.
45. Peeters CM, Leijs MJ, Reijman M, et al. Safety of intra-articular cell-therapy with culture-expanded stem cells in humans: a systematic literature review. Osteoarthritis Cartilage 2013;21(10):1465–73.
46. Marks PW, Witten CM, Califf RM. Clarifying stem-cell therapy's benefits and risks. N Engl J Med 2017;376(11):1007–9.
47. Sekiya I, Muneta T, Horie M, et al. Arthroscopic transplantation of synovial stem cells improves clinical outcomes in knees with cartilage defects. Clin Orthop Relat Res 2015;473(7):2316–26.
48. FDA. FDA warns about stem cell therapies 2017. Available at: https://www.fda.gov/ForConsumers/ConsumerUpdates/ucm286155.htm2017. Accessed March 19, 2019.
49. Jones IA, Togashi RC, Thomas Vangsness C Jr. The economics and regulation of PRP in the evolving field of orthopedic biologics. Curr Rev Musculoskelet Med 2018;11(4):558–65.
50. Sipp DA-O, Caulfield T, Kaye JA-O, et al. Marketing of unproven stem cell-based interventions: a call to action. Sci Transl Med 2017;9(397) [pii:eaag0426].
51. Turner L, Knoepfler P. Selling stem cells in the USA: assessing the direct-to-consumer industry. Cell Stem Cell 2016;19(2):154–7.
52. Piuzzi NS, Ng M, Chughtai M, et al. The stem-cell market for the treatment of knee osteoarthritis: a patient perspective. J Knee Surg 2018;31(6):551–6.
53. Piuzzi NS, Ng M, Kantor A, et al. What is the price and claimed efficacy of platelet-rich plasma injections for the treatment of knee osteoarthritis in the United States? J Knee Surg 2018. https://doi.org/10.1055/s-0038-1669953.
54. DeFrancesco L. California cracks down on stem cell cowboys. Nat Biotechnol 2017;35:1119.
55. Beitzel K, Allen D, Apostolakos J, et al. US definitions, current use, and FDA stance on use of platelet-rich plasma in sports medicine. J Knee Surg 2015;28(1):29–34.
56. Mendick R, Hall A. Europe's largest stem cell clinic shut down after death of baby. The Telegraph 2011. Available at: https://www.telegraph.co.uk. Accessed March 19, 2019.
57. Forsyth J. Three arrested for peddling miracle stem cell cure. Reuters 2012. Available at: https://www.reuters.com. Accessed March 19, 2019.
58. Ramkumar PN, Navarro SM, Haeberle HS, et al. Cellular therapy injections in today's orthopedic market: a social media analysis. Cytotherapy 2017;19(12):1392–9.

Intra-articular Hyaluronan Therapy for Symptomatic Knee Osteoarthritis

Carrie Richardson, MD, MHS*, Anna Plaas, PhD, Joel A. Block, MD

KEYWORDS

• Intra-articular • Hyaluronan • Corticosteroids • Knee osteoarthritis • Pain

KEY POINTS

- Despite numerous randomized controlled trials and meta-analyses of intra-articular hyaluronan therapy (IAHA) for painful knee osteoarthritis, this therapy remains controversial.
- There is a large total treatment benefit of IAHA, the majority of which is mediated by the placebo effect.
- IAHA has small benefits of questionable clinical significance over intra-articular placebo for knee osteoarthritis.
- IAHA is most likely at least comparable to intra-articular corticosteroids for long-term pain relief and may be inferior to intra-articular corticosteroids for short-term pain relief.

INTRODUCTION

Approximately 50% of adults in the United States experience symptoms of knee osteoarthritis over the course of a lifetime,[1] and there is no known pharmacologic therapy that can reverse or prevent its progression. For those affected, knee osteoarthritis has a substantial impact on quality of life as well as work productivity.[2,3] Although knee replacement may be an effective therapy for many, this is a major surgical procedure with 30-day mortality of 1 in 500[4] that requires significant postoperative rehabilitation. Furthermore, many patients either do not want knee arthroplasty or are not appropriate candidates. Therefore, nonsurgical options are essential for the management of the symptoms of knee osteoarthritis. Intra-articular injection of hyaluronan (HA), previously referred to as hyaluronic acid, is a commonly used but controversial nonsurgical therapy for knee osteoarthritis.

Disclosures: Ferring Pharmaceuticals (Dr A. Plaas).
Support: R Katz-J&P Rubschlager Endowmentfor OA Research (Dr A. Plaas).
Department of Internal Medicine, Division of Rheumatology, Rush University Medical Center, Chicago, IL, USA
* Corresponding author. Division of Rheumatology, 1611 West Harrison Street, Suite 510, Chicago, IL 60612.
E-mail address: carrie_richardson@rush.edu

Rheum Dis Clin N Am 45 (2019) 439–451
https://doi.org/10.1016/j.rdc.2019.04.011

Major organizations that represent clinicians and scientists interested in OA therapeutics disagree regarding the appropriateness of intra-articular HA therapy (IAHA), or viscosupplementation, in clinical practice. Osteoarthritis Research Society International guidelines (2014) classified IAHA as "uncertain" for knee osteoarthritis based on selected systematic reviews and meta-analyses,[5] and 2013 guidelines from the American Academy of Orthopaedic Surgeons recommended against IAHA.[6] Despite these guidelines, however, clinicians still commonly recommend IAHA for management of mild to moderate knee osteoarthritis.[7] Furthermore, even as the proportion of newly diagnosed knee osteoarthritis patients receiving IAHA decreased in the decade leading up to the writing of the aforementioned guidelines, the average number of HA injections per patient doubled in the same time period.[8,9] This discrepancy suggests that there are widespread perceived benefits from IAHA among both clinicians and patients.

This article reviews the evidence regarding the use of IAHA for management of knee osteoarthritis. IAHA has been found superior to intra-articular placebo for relief of knee osteoarthritis symptoms in several randomized, placebo-controlled clinical trials,[10–27] and multiple preparations have been approved for use in knee osteoarthritis by the United States Food and Drug Administration (FDA). Overall, however, the incremental benefits of IAHA compared with intra-articular placebo seem small. Furthermore, other randomized controlled studies have failed to detect statistically significant benefits of IAHA compared with intra-articular placebo.[10,22,28–35] Therefore, there is ongoing controversy regarding the benefit provided by IAHA. For any therapy, however, the total treatment effect experienced by the patient includes whatever benefit may be provided by the placebo, which in osteoarthritis pain tends to be substantial.[36] Therefore, the real-world effectiveness of IAHA is greater than what may be inferred based on the small to modest incremental benefits over intra-articular placebo in clinical trials.

In comparison with intra-articular corticosteroids, which generally are less costly, the late benefits of IAHA for pain are most likely at least comparable.[37–45] There may be early benefits, however, of intra-articular corticosteroids compared with IAHA with regard to pain.[44] Although the lower costs of intra-articular corticosteroids and the possible early benefit of corticosteroids over IAHA often are used to argue against IAHA for treatment of knee osteoarthritis, both are effective therapies. Importantly, many patients with knee osteoarthritis are not appropriate candidates for or have not responded favorably to intra-articular corticosteroid injections. In this highly morbid disease with no known disease-modifying therapy, IAHA may be appropriate for some patient groups.

BIOLOGICAL RATIONALE

HA is a high-molecular-weight polysaccharide extracellular matrix molecule with diverse functions in development, growth, and tissue regeneration.[46–49] As a polymer, HA may directly regulate downstream signaling and modulate inflammatory gene expression via cell surface receptors, such as CD44, RHAMM, and Toll-like receptors.[50] It is synthesized at the cell membrane as a protein-free polysaccharide by a set of HA synthases. After its release from the enzyme, it can associated with its receptors or diffuse into the extracellular matrix, where it forms complexes with specific binding proteins that exert various biological effects.[51] For example, HA forms large complexes with aggrecan, versican, and link protein, and these complexes contribute to the structural integrity of cartilage and blood vessels.[47] The individual polymers also may form cross-linked matrices by incorporation of inter-alpha-trypsin–associated heavy chains and pentraxin, catalyzed by TSG6. Such macromolecular complexes have been shown to regular migration and adhesion of inflammatory cells and influence their proinflammatory or anti-inflammatory signaling.[52]

In preclinical animal models of osteoarthritis, IAHA demonstrates beneficial effects on joint tissue integrity as well as pain behaviors. In mice, a single dose of IAHA prevents synovial inflammation and fibrosis, reduces cartilage fibrillation, and decreases early pain sensitization.[53,54] In both mouse and rabbit models of osteoarthritis, IAHA promotes a chrondrogenic response and represses fibrogenenic genes.[55,56] In mice, IAHA also may affect the remodeling of the underlying subchondral bone.[57]

In humans with knee osteoarthritis, some studies have suggested that HA might improve the mechanical properties of the joint and protect against cartilage damage, although this is controversial. Both the viscosity and the HA concentration of knee synovial fluid are reduced in patients with osteoarthritis compared with normal controls.[58,59] In addition, IAHA increases complex shear modulus, which protects against rotational strain, in human knee synovial fluid at 3 months.[60] HA concentration in synovial fluid, however, decreases by approximately 10% per decade, so the decrease in HA concentration associated with osteoarthritis may be related more closely to age than to osteoarthritis.[61] With regard to the theorized chrondroprotective effects of IAHA, early investigations suggested that IAHA may increase chondrocyte density and function in patients with knee osteoarthritis.[62,63] Large clinical trials, however, have in general failed to demonstrate a clinically significant structure-modifying effect, and these possible histological changes are of unclear significance. Furthermore, the mechanisms by which IAHA may reduce pain sensation remain poorly understood.

INTRA-ARTICULAR HYALURONAN PREPARATIONS AND ADMINISTRATION

The first HA products for intra-articular injection were purified from rooster comb, but genetically engineered bacteria containing HA synthase are now used to produce large amounts of the polymer through fermentation processes. Injectable HA preparations may vary in molecular weight (approximately 1 million molecular weight) and in degree of chemically introduced cross-linking. Chemically cross-linked products have a longer half-life in the joint space after injection and exert longer-lasting biological or biophysical effects in the joint. A previous study suggested that lower-molecular-weight single-chain preparations may be less effective than higher-molecular-weight preparations in relieving pain and stiffness,[64] but this result has not been confirmed.

There are numerous FDA-approved preparations of HA for intra-articular injection. These HA products vary widely in price and administration schedules (**Table 1**). With regard to cost, it is difficult to estimate actual patient expense because of variations in pricing by geography, insurance status, and other factors. The average wholesaler acquisition cost for a single treatment course, however, averages approximately $1000, not including the associated costs of the clinic visits and injection procedures. With regard to administration schedule, depending on the HA preparation used, a single treatment course may consist of a single intra-articular injection or a series of 3 to 5 weekly injections.

Adverse effects of IAHA preparations have been reported, particularly with cross-linked products, and typically consist of joint pain and inflammation.[65,66] In a study of 1 cross-linked product, nonanimal stabilized hyaluronic acid (NASHA), versus intra-articular corticosteroids, patients treated with NASHA in the blinded phase were approximately 5 times more likely to have arthralgia than patients treated with

Table 1
Food and Drug Administration–approved hyaluronan preparations for osteoarthritis of the knee

Product	Source	Size, Characteristics	Weekly Injections	Cost[a]
Durolane (Bioventus)	Bacterial	High molecular weight: NASHA cross-linked	1	$975.00
Euflexxa (Ferring)	Bacterial	2.4–3.6 × 106 kDa	3	$1019.00
Gel-One (Zimmer Biomet)	Chicken comb	High-molecular-weight cross-linked dimers	1	$998.00
GelSyn-3 (Bioventus)	Bacterial	1100 kDa	3	$1035.00
GenVisc 850 (OrthogenRx)	Bacterial	620–1170 kDa	5	$1350.00
Hyalgan (Sanofi-Aventis; Fidia)	Chicken comb	500–730 kDa	3 or 5	$950.00
Hymovis (Fidia)	Bacterial	500–730 kDa	2	$872.00
Monovisc (DePuy)	Bacterial	1000–2900 kDa, cross-linked	1	$1360.00
Orthovisc (DePuy Mitek)	Chicken comb	1100–2900 kDa	3 or 4	$1368.00
Supartz/Supartz FX (Smith & Nephew)	Chicken comb	620–1170 kDa	3 or 5	$1151.50
Synojoynt (Teva)	Not specified	2500 kDa	3	NA
Synvisc (Synvisc-One) (Genzyme Biosurgery)	Chicken comb	>6000 kDa cross-linked hylans	3 (1)	$1284.10
TriVisc (OrthogenRx)	Bacterial	Not specified	3	NA
Visco-3 (Zimmer Biomet; Bioventus)	Chicken comb	620–1170 kDa	3	$750.00

Abbreviation: NA, not available.
[a] Average wholesaler acquisition cost for 1 dosage regimen.
Adapted from Two new intra-articular injections for knee osteoarthritis. Med Lett Drugs Ther 2018 Aug 27;60(1554):142–144; with permission.

the comparator.[67] Acute pseudoseptic arthritis reactions have been associated with hylan G-F 20, a high-molecular-weight cross-linked product, particularly with repeated courses of therapy.[68] Pseudoseptic reactions are rare but frequently result in hospitalization when they occur. Both acute gout[69] and acute pseudogout[70] also have been described as complicating IAHA.

Importantly, IAHA may not be acceptable to patients who avoid animal-based products. Even products that are made by biofermentation, however, may use animal products in the growth media. Clinicians should consider counseling patients regarding the animal-based nature of many of these products prior to injection.

THE PLACEBO EFFECT IN INTRA-ARTICULAR THERAPY

A nuanced understanding of the placebo effect is critical for interpreting the results of osteoarthritis clinical trials, because there is a striking discrepancy between the small to modest incremental benefits of IAHA over placebo seen in clinical trials and the substantial real-world effectiveness of this therapy. First, what is often referred to as the "placebo effect" is a complex phenomenon that incorporates not only the vehicle but also the contextual effects, including the environment in which the treatment is delivered and patient expectations regarding the benefit of the treatment.[71,72] Contextual effects, for example, may be enhanced when a patient sees an operating room with high-tech equipment, even if the equipment is not used to deliver the intervention. Contextual effects also may be enhanced when a patient has confidence in the doctor administering the treatment or when a patient perceives a therapy as innovative. The contextual effect varies widely but may account for 75% of the overall treatment effect in randomized controlled trials of osteoarthritis pain.[36]

As intra-articular therapy is more invasive and, therefore, inspires greater patient and provider expectations than oral therapy; intra-articular therapy generally is more effective than oral therapy.[64,73] This results in smaller benefits of IAHA when IAHA is compared with intra-articular placebo as opposed to when IAHA is compared with oral placebo (**Fig. 1**). Bannuru and colleagues[74] quantified this effect, demonstrating that comparison of IAHA to intra-articular placebo as opposed to oral placebo reduces the benefits of IAHA by about half. The placebo effect also can vary, however, depending on the active intra-articular treatment, and the placebo effect of intra-articular saline is larger in trials of IAHA than in trials of intra-articular corticosteroid.[73,75] Other factors that may enhance the placebo effect include prohibiting the use of rescue medications as well as larger sample sizes.[73] Surprisingly, the placebo effect can be a durable phenomenon in osteoarthritis clinical trials, persisting for as long as 6 months to 12 months.[75]

Placebo and contextual effects are particularly evident in uncontrolled trials and epidemiologic studies, which demonstrate substantial benefits of IAHA. For example, in an early open-label study by Namiki and colleagues,[76] approximately three-fourths of patients treated with IAHA demonstrated improvement in knee pain and function. In addition, Quilliot and colleagues[77] examined survey data from 166 patients and found that 71% of the survey responders reported improvement at 3 months, and 78% reported improvement at 6 months. Because of the substantial placebo and contextual effects in trials of osteoarthritis pain, however, results of these and other uncontrolled studies need to be interpreted carefully.

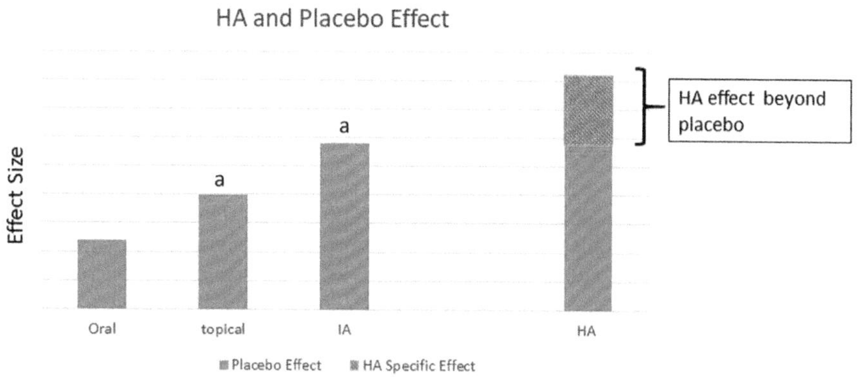

Fig. 1. The effect size of placebo increases with the invasiveness of the delivery. Topical placebo has a significantly higher effect size than oral and intra-articular is higher than topical. The placebo effect accounts for more than 70% of the total therapeutic effect of HA. [a] statistically significant. (*Data from* Bannuru RR, McAlindon TE, Sullivan MC, Wong JB, Kent DM, Schmid CH. Effectiveness and implications of alternative placebo treatments: a systematic review and network meta-analysis of osteoarthritis trials. *Annals of internal medicine.* Sep 1 2015;163(5):365–37; and Zou K, Wong J, Abdullah N, et al. Examination of overall treatment effect and the proportion attributable to contextual effect in osteoarthritis: meta-analysis of randomised controlled trials. *Annals of the rheumatic diseases.* Nov 2016;75(11):1964–1970)

RANDOMIZED CONTROLLED TRIALS AND META-ANALYSES OF RANDOMIZED CONTROLLED TRIALS

A large number of randomized controlled trials, meta-analyses of randomized controlled trials, and even a systematic review of meta-analyses of randomized controlled trials[78] have been published on the subjected of IAHA. Randomized controlled trials and meta-analyses of IAHA vary widely, however, in methodological quality, and there is considerable debate about the results of these studies.

With regard to the systematic reviews and meta-analyses, these studies are subject to several serious methodological issues. For example, there often is substantial methodological heterogeneity in the randomized controlled trials included in the meta-analyses. Therefore, it may not be appropriate to pool the results into an overall effect estimate despite acceptable I^2 values for heterogeneity. For example, some studies may include more patients with late-stage knee osteoarthritis, which may be less likely to respond to IAHA than earlier-stage knee osteoarthritis.[79] In addition, several meta-analyses include studies with inadequate blinding, which may introduce considerable bias and skew the results in favor of the active treatment. In a meta-analysis with few studies, the results from 1 low-quality study with inadequate blinding may dramatically change the overall effect estimate.

Despite varying methodologies and analytical methods, however, randomized controlled trials and meta-analyses overall demonstrate a benefit of IAHA over placebo. A Cochrane review demonstrated a moderate to large benefit of IAHA compared with placebo, an effect that peaks at 5 weeks to 13 weeks after the injection.[43] Another systematic review and meta-analysis of osteoarthritis clinical trials also demonstrated significant benefits of IAHA acid versus intra-articular placebo.[74] Nevertheless, there is ongoing debate about the clinical importance of these benefits over intra-articular therapy. Vannabouathong and colleagues[64] found that, after including the effects of intra-articular placebo compared with oral placebo (0.29 standardized mean difference), there were clinically important benefits of higher-molecular-weight HA preparations (≥1500 kD) compared with placebo. The clinical importance of the pain benefit of IAHA over placebo, however, remains questionable.

Although there is a clear incremental benefit of questionable clinical significance of IAHA over intra-articular placebo, IAHA may be no better than intra-articular corticosteroids with regard to pain. Consistent with understanding of the placebo effect in osteoarthritis trials, open-label and inadequately blinded studies demonstrate a greater benefit of IAHA over intra-articular corticosteroids.[80,81] In contrast, however, well-designed studies with adequate blinding demonstrate a lack of significant difference in patient-reported outcomes between IAHA and intra-articular corticosteroids. For example, in a multicenter randomized trial of intra-articular corticosteroids versus IAHA that evaluated 391 patients, there were no significant differences in Western Ontario and McMaster Universities Osteoarthritis Index (WOMAC) pain scores at any time point during the 6-month treatment period.[38] In another multicenter randomized trial of 442 patients, there were no significant differences in WOMAC pain responder rates between the IAHA and intra-articular corticosteroid groups throughout the 26-week blinded phase.[67]

In contrast to the aforementioned trials, some clinical trials and meta-analyses of IAHA versus intra-articular corticosteroids have suggested differential benefits of either therapy according to length of follow-up, with a possible early benefit of intra-articular corticosteroids and a later benefit of IAHA. For example, an open-label study by Leardini and colleagues[81] demonstrated that pain scores improved similarly in both the IAHA and the intra-articular corticosteroid treatment groups until 21 days after the initiation of treatment. Subsequently, the hyaluronic acid group had superior pain relief. In an adequately blinded study of 110 patients conducted in Thailand, however, an early benefit of intra-articular corticosteroids compared with IAHA was observed with regard to both visual analog scale (VAS) pain scores and WOMAC scores within the first 2 weeks, but benefits of each therapy were similar at 6 months.[40] Similar results were reported in an Iranian study of 140 patients, in which intra-articular corticosteroids seemed superior to IAHA in the first month, but the advantage disappeared by 3 months.[42] Similarly, a meta-analysis that included inadequately blinded and open-label studies concluded that IAHA was superior to intra-articular corticosteroids at 3 months and 6 months but not at 1 month.[45] A subsequent meta-analysis that included many of the same studies reported that IAHA was inferior to intra-articular corticosteroids at 1 month and had no advantage at 3 months.[44] Similar to the previous analysis, however, this meta-analysis concluded that IAHA had significant advantage over intra-articular corticosteroids at 6 months.

Considering the possible early benefit of intra-articular corticosteroids and the possible late benefit of IAHA, combination therapy with IAHA as well as corticosteroids recently has been studied. In a randomized trial of 40 patients in Turkey, patients receiving IAHA acid plus intra-articular corticosteroids had greater reductions in pain at 1 month compared with patients receiving IAHA alone.[82] This study, however, was not adequately blinded. A randomized controlled trial of 120 patients in China with adequate blinding demonstrated statistically significant benefits of intra-articular corticosteroid plus HA over IAHA alone with regard to VAS pain and WOMAC pain in the first 3 months of therapy.[83] In a 3-arm randomized, multicenter trial of 98 patients, Petrella and colleagues[84] demonstrated similar reductions in WOMAC pain, stiffness, and function scores of 30% to 50% at 26 weeks in the intra-articular HA plus corticosteroid group compared with either of the other IAHA groups.

In summary, IAHA is better than intra-articular placebo for relieving pain from knee osteoarthritis, although the clinical significance of this benefit is unclear. When compared with intra-articular corticosteroids, IAHA may be inferior for pain relief within the first month but comparable or superior at 3 months to 6 months. The efficacy of combination therapy with both intra-articular corticosteroids and IAHA is still unproved.

INTRA-ARTICULAR HYALURONAN THERAPY AND KNEE ARTHROPLASTY

The pain relief and improved knee function observed with IAHA may result in significant delay or deferral of surgery. Knee arthroplasty is a major procedure with associated morbidity and mortality as well as an average cost of $30,000 in the United States according to Blue Cross Blue Shield estimates.[85] This price, however, does not include the requisite costs for rehabilitation, physical therapy, days lost from work, outpatient clinic visits, and personal care expenses during surgical recovery. Hence, presumably avoidance or deferral of knee arthroplasty would be desirable. Although time to arthroplasty is a difficult outcome to assess in clinical trials of short duration, epidemiologic and retrospective data suggest that there may be a benefit to the use of IAHA with regard to delay of knee arthroplasty.[86] In an analysis of the 5% Part B Medicare Data (2005–2012) restricted to patients who had undergone knee replacement, IAHA was associated with delayed arthroplasty of 9 months compared with no IAHA.[87] Another study that used a 10% sample of LifeLink Plus claims from 2010 to 2015 and restricted the analysis to patients who received surgery demonstrated a statistically significant reduction in the hazard of knee arthroplasty of 13% to 14% in patients who had received IAHA compared with either patients who received intra-articular corticosteroids or patients who received no IAHA and no intra-articular corticosteroids.[88]

SUMMARY

IAHA has substantial effects in clinical practice but only small to modest incremental benefits over intra-articular placebo in high-quality clinical trials. This discrepancy is due in large part to the placebo effect, which is considerable in trials of osteoarthritis pain. Although the majority of the benefit of IAHA for osteoarthritis pain is due to the placebo effect, there remains a significant and possibly clinically important additive benefit of IAHA over intra-articular placebo. Furthermore, IAHA clearly is effective in a significant number of patients in clinical practice, even if the majority of the benefit is not due to the active drug.

There is a substantial unmet medical need for effective medical options to treat osteoarthritis pain. Although intra-articular corticosteroids may be less costly than IAHA,[89] there are many patients who fail intra-articular corticosteroid therapy and who may benefit from IAHA. Although IAHA preparations may cost approximately $1000 per cycle, this is considerably less than the cost of a total knee arthroplasty. Furthermore, the adverse effects of IAHA generally are mild and self-limited. Overall, IAHA may be an appropriate and effective therapy in patients with symptomatic knee osteoarthritis.

REFERENCES

1. Murphy L, Schwartz TA, Helmick CG, et al. Lifetime risk of symptomatic knee osteoarthritis. Arthritis Rheum 2008;59(9):1207–13.
2. Agaliotis M, Fransen M, Bridgett L, et al. Risk factors associated with reduced work productivity among people with chronic knee pain. Osteoarthritis Cartilage 2013;21(9):1160–9.
3. Hoogeboom TJ, den Broeder AA, de Bie RA, et al. Longitudinal impact of joint pain comorbidity on quality of life and activity levels in knee osteoarthritis: data from the osteoarthritis initiative. Rheumatology 2013;52(3):543–6.
4. Berstock JR, Beswick AD, Lopez-Lopez JA, et al. Mortality after total knee arthroplasty: a systematic review of incidence, temporal trends, and risk factors. J Bone Joint Surg Am 2018;100(12):1064–70.
5. McAlindon TE, Bannuru RR, Sullivan MC, et al. OARSI guidelines for the non-surgical management of knee osteoarthritis. Osteoarthritis Cartilage 2014;22(3):363–88.
6. Directors AAoOSBo. Treatment of osteoarthritis of the knee. Evidence-based guideline. 1st edition 2008.
7. Carlson VR, Ong AC, Orozco FR, et al. Compliance with the AAOS guidelines for treatment of osteoarthritis of the knee: a survey of the American Association of Hip and Knee Surgeons. J Am Acad Orthop Surg 2018;26(3):103–7.
8. Koenig KM, Ong KL, Lau EC, et al. The use of hyaluronic acid and corticosteroid injections among medicare patients with knee osteoarthritis. J Arthroplasty 2016;31(2):351–5.
9. Bedard NA, DeMik DE, Glass NA, et al. Impact of clinical practice guidelines on use of intra-articular hyaluronic acid and corticosteroid injections for knee osteoarthritis. J Bone Joint Surg Am 2018;100(10):827–34.
10. Dixon AS, Jacoby RK, Berry H, et al. Clinical trial of intra-articular injection of sodium hyaluronate in patients with osteoarthritis of the knee. Curr Med Res Opin 1988;11(4):205–13.

11. Dougados M, Nguyen M, Listrat V, et al. High molecular weight sodium hyaluronate (hyalectin) in osteoarthritis of the knee: a 1 year placebo-controlled trial. Osteoarthritis Cartilage 1993;1(2):97–103.
12. Altman RD, Moskowitz R. Intraarticular sodium hyaluronate (Hyalgan) in the treatment of patients with osteoarthritis of the knee: a randomized clinical trial. Hyalgan Study Group. J Rheumatol 1998;25(11):2203–12.
13. Huskisson EC, Donnelly S. Hyaluronic acid in the treatment of osteoarthritis of the knee. Rheumatology 1999;38(7):602–7.
14. Kotevoglu N, Iyibozkurt PC, Hiz O, et al. A prospective randomised controlled clinical trial comparing the efficacy of different molecular weight hyaluronan solutions in the treatment of knee osteoarthritis. Rheumatol Int 2006;26(4):325–30.
15. Petrella RJ, Petrella M. A prospective, randomized, double-blind, placebo controlled study to evaluate the efficacy of intraarticular hyaluronic acid for osteoarthritis of the knee. J Rheumatol 2006;33(5):951–6.
16. Petrella RJ, Cogliano A, Decaria J. Combining two hyaluronic acids in osteoarthritis of the knee: a randomized, double-blind, placebo-controlled trial. Clin Rheumatol 2008;27(8):975–81.
17. Chevalier X, Jerosch J, Goupille P, et al. Single, intra-articular treatment with 6 ml hylan G-F 20 in patients with symptomatic primary osteoarthritis of the knee: a randomised, multicentre, double-blind, placebo controlled trial. Ann Rheum Dis 2010;69(1):113–9.
18. Kul-Panza E, Berker N. Is hyaluronate sodium effective in the management of knee osteoarthritis? A placebo-controlled double-blind study. Minerva Med 2010;101(2):63–72.
19. Navarro-Sarabia F, Coronel P, Collantes E, et al. A 40-month multicentre, randomised placebo-controlled study to assess the efficacy and carry-over effect of repeated intra-articular injections of hyaluronic acid in knee osteoarthritis: the AMELIA project. Ann Rheum Dis 2011;70(11):1957–62.
20. Huang TL, Chang CC, Lee CH, et al. Intra-articular injections of sodium hyaluronate (Hyalgan(R)) in osteoarthritis of the knee. a randomized, controlled, double-blind, multicenter trial in the Asian population. BMC Musculoskelet Disord 2011; 12:221.
21. DeCaria JE, Montero-Odasso M, Wolfe D, et al. The effect of intra-articular hyaluronic acid treatment on gait velocity in older knee osteoarthritis patients: a randomized, controlled study. Arch Gerontol Geriatr 2012;55(2):310–5.
22. Arden NK, Akermark C, Andersson M, et al. A randomized saline-controlled trial of NASHA hyaluronic acid for knee osteoarthritis. Curr Med Res Opin 2014;30(2): 279–86.
23. Wu JJ, Shih LY, Hsu HC, et al. The double-blind test of sodium hyaluronate (ARTZ) on osteoarthritis knee. Zhonghua yi xue za zhi 1997;59(2):99–106.
24. Tamir E, Robinson D, Koren R, et al. Intra-articular hyaluronan injections for the treatment of osteoarthritis of the knee: a randomized, double blind, placebo controlled study. Clin Exp Rheumatol 2001;19(3):265–70.
25. Petrella RJ, DiSilvestro MD, Hildebrand C. Effects of hyaluronate sodium on pain and physical functioning in osteoarthritis of the knee: a randomized, double-blind, placebo-controlled clinical trial. Arch Intern Med 2002;162(3):292–8.
26. Karlsson J, Sjogren LS, Lohmander LS. Comparison of two hyaluronan drugs and placebo in patients with knee osteoarthritis. A controlled, randomized, double-blind, parallel-design multicentre study. Rheumatology 2002;41(11):1240–8.

27. Cubukcu D, Ardic F, Karabulut N, et al. Hylan G-F 20 efficacy on articular cartilage quality in patients with knee osteoarthritis: clinical and MRI assessment. Clin Rheumatol 2005;24(4):336–41.
28. Jorgensen A, Stengaard-Pedersen K, Simonsen O, et al. Intra-articular hyaluronan is without clinical effect in knee osteoarthritis: a multicentre, randomised, placebo-controlled, double-blind study of 337 patients followed for 1 year. Ann Rheum Dis 2010;69(6):1097–102.
29. Creamer P, Sharif M, George E, et al. Intra-articular hyaluronic acid in osteoarthritis of the knee: an investigation into mechanisms of action. Osteoarthritis Cartilage 1994;2(2):133–40.
30. Henderson EB, Smith EC, Pegley F, et al. Intra-articular injections of 750 kD hyaluronan in the treatment of osteoarthritis: a randomised single centre double-blind placebo-controlled trial of 91 patients demonstrating lack of efficacy. Ann Rheum Dis 1994;53(8):529–34.
31. Lohmander LS, Dalen N, Englund G, et al. Intra-articular hyaluronan injections in the treatment of osteoarthritis of the knee: a randomised, double blind, placebo controlled multicentre trial. Hyaluronan Multicentre Trial Group. Ann Rheum Dis 1996;55(7):424–31.
32. Altman RD, Akermark C, Beaulieu AD, et al. Efficacy and safety of a single intra-articular injection of non-animal stabilized hyaluronic acid (NASHA) in patients with osteoarthritis of the knee. Osteoarthritis Cartilage 2004;12(8):642–9.
33. Pham T, Le Henanff A, Ravaud P, et al. Evaluation of the symptomatic and structural efficacy of a new hyaluronic acid compound, NRD101, in comparison with diacerein and placebo in a 1 year randomised controlled study in symptomatic knee osteoarthritis. Ann Rheum Dis 2004;63(12):1611–7.
34. Lundsgaard C, Dufour N, Fallentin E, et al. Intra-articular sodium hyaluronate 2 mL versus physiological saline 20 mL versus physiological saline 2 mL for painful knee osteoarthritis: a randomized clinical trial. Scand J Rheumatol 2008;37(2):142–50.
35. van der Weegen W, Wullems JA, Bos E, et al. No difference between intra-articular injection of hyaluronic acid and placebo for mild to moderate knee osteoarthritis: a randomized, controlled, double-blind trial. J Arthroplasty 2015;30(5):754–7.
36. Zou K, Wong J, Abdullah N, et al. Examination of overall treatment effect and the proportion attributable to contextual effect in osteoarthritis: meta-analysis of randomised controlled trials. Ann Rheum Dis 2016;75(11):1964–70.
37. Shimizu M, Higuchi H, Takagishi K, et al. Clinical and biochemical characteristics after intra-articular injection for the treatment of osteoarthritis of the knee: prospective randomized study of sodium hyaluronate and corticosteroid. J Orthop Sci 2010;15(1):51–6.
38. Housman L, Arden N, Schnitzer TJ, et al. Intra-articular hylastan versus steroid for knee osteoarthritis. Knee Surg Sports Traumatol Arthrosc 2014;22(7):1684–92.
39. Bisicchia S, Bernardi G, Tudisco C. HYADD 4 versus methylprednisolone acetate in symptomatic knee osteoarthritis: a single-centre single blind prospective randomised controlled clinical study with 1-year follow-up. Clin Exp Rheumatol 2016;34(5):857–63.
40. Tammachote N, Kanitnate S, Yakumpor T, et al. Intra-articular, single-shot hylan G-F 20 hyaluronic acid injection compared with corticosteroid in knee osteoarthritis: a double-blind, randomized controlled trial. J Bone Joint Surg Am 2016;98(11):885–92.

41. Campos ALS, RSP EA, da Silva EB, et al. Viscosupplementation in patients with severe osteoarthritis of the knee: six month follow-up of a randomized, double-blind clinical trial. Int Orthop 2017;41(11):2273–80.
42. Askari A, Gholami T, NaghiZadeh MM, et al. Hyaluronic acid compared with corticosteroid injections for the treatment of osteoarthritis of the knee: a randomized control trail. SpringerPlus 2016;5:442.
43. Bellamy N. Hyaluronic acid and knee osteoarthritis. J Fam Pract 2006;55(11): 967–8.
44. He WW, Kuang MJ, Zhao J, et al. Efficacy and safety of intraarticular hyaluronic acid and corticosteroid for knee osteoarthritis: a meta-analysis. Int J Surg 2017; 39:95–103.
45. Wang F, He X. Intra-articular hyaluronic acid and corticosteroids in the treatment of knee osteoarthritis: a meta-analysis. Exp Ther Med 2015;9(2):493–500.
46. Schmidt TA, Gastelum NS, Nguyen QT, et al. Boundary lubrication of articular cartilage: role of synovial fluid constituents. Arthritis Rheum 2007;56(3):882–91.
47. Culav EM, Clark CH, Merrilees MJ. Connective tissues: matrix composition and its relevance to physical therapy. Phys Ther 1999;79(3):308–19.
48. Canoso JJ, Stack MT, Brandt KD. Hyaluronic acid content of deep and subcutaneous bursae of man. Ann Rheum Dis 1983;42(2):171–5.
49. Cowman MK, Schmidt TA, Raghavan P, et al. Viscoelastic properties of hyaluronan in physiological conditions. F1000Res 2015;4:622.
50. Dicker KT, Gurski LA, Pradhan-Bhatt S, et al. Hyaluronan: a simple polysaccharide with diverse biological functions. Acta Biomater 2014;10(4):1558–70.
51. Day AJ. The structure and regulation of hyaluronan-binding proteins. Biochem Soc Trans 1999;27(2):115–21.
52. Wisniewski HG, Burgess WH, Oppenheim JD, et al. TSG-6, an arthritis-associated hyaluronan binding protein, forms a stable complex with the serum protein inter-alpha-inhibitor. Biochemistry 1994;33(23):7423–9.
53. Plaas A, Li J, Riesco J, et al. Intraarticular injection of hyaluronan prevents cartilage erosion, periarticular fibrosis and mechanical allodynia and normalizes stance time in murine knee osteoarthritis. Arthritis Res Ther 2011;13(2):R46.
54. Muramatsu Y, Sasho T, Saito M, et al. Preventive effects of hyaluronan from deterioration of gait parameters in surgically induced mice osteoarthritic knee model. Osteoarthritis Cartilage 2014;22(6):831–5.
55. Li J, Gorski DJ, Anemaet W, et al. Hyaluronan injection in murine osteoarthritis prevents TGFbeta 1-induced synovial neovascularization and fibrosis and maintains articular cartilage integrity by a CD44-dependent mechanism. Arthritis Res Ther 2012;14(3):R151.
56. Kaderli S, Viguier E, Watrelot-Virieux D, et al. Efficacy study of two novel hyaluronic acid-based formulations for viscosupplementation therapy in an early osteoarthrosic rabbit model. Eur J Pharm Biopharm 2015;96:388–95.
57. Quan Shen Q, LJ, Chan D, et al. Effect of intra-articular hyaluronan injection on inflammation and bone remodeling in the epiphyses and metaphyses of the knee in a murine model of joint injury. Am J Transl Res, in press.
58. Stafford CT, Niedermeier W, Holley HL, et al. Studies on the concentration and intrinsic viscosity of hyaluronic acid in synovial fluids of patients with rheumatic diseases. Ann Rheum Dis 1964;23:152–7.
59. Dahl LB, Dahl IM, Engstrom-Laurent A, et al. Concentration and molecular weight of sodium hyaluronate in synovial fluid from patients with rheumatoid arthritis and other arthropathies. Ann Rheum Dis 1985;44(12):817–22.

60. Bagga H, Burkhardt D, Sambrook P, et al. Longterm effects of intraarticular hyaluronan on synovial fluid in osteoarthritis of the knee. J Rheumatol 2006;33(5):946–50.
61. Temple-Wong MM, Ren S, Quach P, et al. Hyaluronan concentration and size distribution in human knee synovial fluid: variations with age and cartilage degeneration. Arthritis Res Ther 2016;18:18.
62. Frizziero L, Govoni E, Bacchini P. Intra-articular hyaluronic acid in the treatment of osteoarthritis of the knee: clinical and morphological study. Clin Exp Rheumatol 1998;16(4):441–9.
63. Guidolin DD, Ronchetti IP, Lini E, et al. Morphological analysis of articular cartilage biopsies from a randomized, clinical study comparing the effects of 500-730 kDa sodium hyaluronate (Hyalgan) and methylprednisolone acetate on primary osteoarthritis of the knee. Osteoarthritis Cartilage 2001;9(4):371–81.
64. Vannabouathong C, Bhandari M, Bedi A, et al. Nonoperative treatments for knee osteoarthritis: an evaluation of treatment characteristics and the intra-articular placebo effect: a systematic review. JBJS Rev 2018;6(7):e5.
65. Martens PB. Bilateral symmetric inflammatory reaction to hylan G-F 20 injection. Arthritis Rheum 2001;44(4):978–9.
66. Kroesen S, Schmid W, Theiler R. Induction of an acute attack of calcium pyrophosphate dihydrate arthritis by intra-articular injection of hylan G-F 20 (Synvisc). Clin Rheumatol 2000;19(2):147–9.
67. Leighton R, Akermark C, Therrien R, et al. NASHA hyaluronic acid vs. methylprednisolone for knee osteoarthritis: a prospective, multi-centre, randomized, non-inferiority trial. Osteoarthritis Cartilage 2014;22(1):17–25.
68. Leopold SS, Warme WJ, Pettis PD, et al. Increased frequency of acute local reaction to intra-articular hylan GF-20 (synvisc) in patients receiving more than one course of treatment. J Bone Joint Surg Am 2002;84-A(9):1619–23.
69. Yacyshyn EA, Matteson EL. Gout after intraarticular injection of hylan GF-20 (Synvisc). J Rheumatol 1999;26(12):2717.
70. Ali Y, Weinstein M, Jokl P. Acute pseudogout following intra-articular injection of high molecular weight hyaluronic acid. Am J Med 1999;107(6):641–2.
71. Zhang W, Zou K, Doherty M. Placebos for knee osteoarthritis: reaffirmation of "needle is better than pill". Ann Intern Med 2015;163(5):392–3.
72. Doherty M, Dieppe P. The "placebo" response in osteoarthritis and its implications for clinical practice. Osteoarthritis Cartilage 2009;17(10):1255–62.
73. Zhang W, Robertson J, Jones AC, et al. The placebo effect and its determinants in osteoarthritis: meta-analysis of randomised controlled trials. Ann Rheum Dis 2008;67(12):1716–23.
74. Bannuru RR, McAlindon TE, Sullivan MC, et al. Effectiveness and implications of alternative placebo treatments: a systematic review and network meta-analysis of osteoarthritis trials. Ann Intern Med 2015;163(5):365–72.
75. Altman RD, Devji T, Bhandari M, et al. Clinical benefit of intra-articular saline as a comparator in clinical trials of knee osteoarthritis treatments: a systematic review and meta-analysis of randomized trials. Semin Arthritis Rheum 2016;46(2):151–9.
76. Namiki O, Toyoshima H, Morisaki N. Therapeutic effect of intra-articular injection of high molecular weight hyaluronic acid on osteoarthritis of the knee. Int J Clin Pharmacol Ther Toxicol 1982;20(11):501–7.
77. Quilliot J, Couderc M, Giraud C, et al. Efficacy of intra-articular hyaluronic acid injection in knee osteoarthritis in everyday life. Semin Arthritis Rheum 2019. [Epub ahead of print].

78. Campbell KA, Erickson BJ, Saltzman BM, et al. Is local viscosupplementation injection clinically superior to other therapies in the treatment of osteoarthritis of the knee: a systematic review of overlapping meta-analyses. Arthroscopy 2015; 31(10):2036–45.e14.
79. Nicholls M, Shaw P, Niazi F, et al. The impact of excluding patients with end-stage knee disease in intra-articular hyaluronic acid trials: a systematic review and meta-analysis. Adv Ther 2019;36(1):147–61.
80. Trueba Davalillo CA, Trueba Vasavilbaso C, Navarrete Alvarez JM, et al. Clinical efficacy of intra-articular injections in knee osteoarthritis: a prospective randomized study comparing hyaluronic acid and betamethasone. Open Access Rheumatol 2015;7:9–18.
81. Leardini G, Mattara L, Franceschini M, et al. Intra-articular treatment of knee osteoarthritis. A comparative study between hyaluronic acid and 6-methyl prednisolone acetate. Clin Exp Rheumatol 1991;9(4):375–81.
82. Ozturk C, Atamaz F, Hepguler S, et al. The safety and efficacy of intraarticular hyaluronan with/without corticosteroid in knee osteoarthritis: 1-year, single-blind, randomized study. Rheumatol Int 2006;26(4):314–9.
83. Wang SZ, Wu DY, Chang Q, et al. Intra-articular, single-shot co-injection of hyaluronic acid and corticosteroids in knee osteoarthritis: A randomized controlled trial. Exp Ther Med 2018;16(3):1928–34.
84. Petrella RJ, Emans PJ, Alleyne J, et al. Safety and performance of Hydros and Hydros-TA for knee osteoarthritis: a prospective, multicenter, randomized, double-blind feasibility trial. BMC Musculoskelet Disord 2015;16:57.
85. Shield BCB. A study of cost variations for knee and hip replacement surgeries in the U.S. 2017.
86. Delbarre A, Amor B, Bardoulat I, et al. Do intra-articular hyaluronic acid injections delay total knee replacement in patients with osteoarthritis - a Cox model analysis. PLoS One 2017;12(11):e0187227.
87. Ong KL, Anderson AF, Niazi F, et al. Hyaluronic acid injections in medicare knee osteoarthritis patients are associated with longer time to knee arthroplasty. J Arthroplasty 2016;31(8):1667–73.
88. Shewale AR, Barnes CL, Fischbach LA, et al. Comparative effectiveness of intra-articular hyaluronic acid and corticosteroid injections on the time to surgical knee procedures. J Arthroplasty 2017;32(12):3591–7.e24.
89. Levin PE. Utilizing health-care resources wisely: understanding the efficacy of our interventions: commentary on an article by Nattapol Tammachote, MD, MSc, et al.: "Intra-articular, single-shot hylan G-F 20 hyaluronic acid injection compared with corticosteroid in knee osteoarthritis. a double-blind, randomized controlled trial". J Bone Joint Surg Am 2016;98(11):e47.

Vascular Consequences of Hyperuricemia and Hypouricemia

Daniel Albert, MD[a,*], Paige N. Scudder, MLIS[b],
Pamela Bagley, PhD, MSLIS[b], Kenneth G. Saag, MD, MSc[c]

KEYWORDS

• Gout • Hyperuricemia • Hypouricemia • Vascular • Atherosclerosis
• Cardiovascular • Cerebrovascular

KEY POINTS

- The question of whether gout and hyperuricemia are risk factors for vascular disease is one of the most controversial areas of rheumatology, with enormous implications for management.
- The authors searched the English-language literature for studies published from 2017 to February 15, 2019, using subject headings and keywords to capture the concepts of hyperuricemia and cardiovascular disease, with a separate search for hypouricemia with the same parameters in addition to a search of published systematic reviews from 1999 to 2019.
- Hyperuricemia has been implicated in a variety of conditions, including hypertension, chronic renal insufficiency, coronary artery disease, myocardial infarction, atherosclerosis, stroke, heart failure, and all-cause mortality.
- There is an abundance of circumstantial evidence associating hyperuricemia and gout to atherosclerosis; however, much of it is confounded by associated comorbidity.
- Overall, the interventional data on both canakinumab and colchicine are a stronger argument for gout as a risk factor for vascular disease than hyperuricemia, but there are some interventional data implicating hyperuricemia in some individuals as a risk factor for hypertension, which might be an indirect mechanism to link hyperuricemia to atherosclerosis.

Disclosure Statement: None.
[a] The Dartmouth Institute, Geisel School of Medicine, Dartmouth-Hitchcock Medical Center, 1 Rope Ferry Road, Hanover, NH 03755, USA; [b] Biomedical Libraries, Dartmouth College, Hanover, NH, USA; [c] Division of Clinical Immunology and Rheumatology, Department of Medicine, University of Alabama Birmingham, 1670 University Boulevard, Birmingham, AL 35233, USA
* Corresponding author.
E-mail address: Daniel.A.Albert@Hitchcock.org

Rheum Dis Clin N Am 45 (2019) 453–464
https://doi.org/10.1016/j.rdc.2019.04.005

INTRODUCTION

The question of whether gout and hyperuricemia are risk factors for vascular disease is one of the most controversial areas of rheumatology. If gout is found to predispose to atherosclerosis, the approach to management will necessarily change from the internists' stance that gout should be treated symptomatically to the rheumatologists' conviction that gout should be managed in a treat-to-target approach. Even more importantly, if hyperuricemia, which is now present in up to one-third of the United States adult population, is found an independent risk factor for vascular disease, then the implications possibly are more wide reaching than the use of statins for hyperlipidemia. This review, with a systematic search, addresses the background and rationale for the urate hypothesis, the possible associations that are based largely on observational data, the implications of those observations, the more recent interventional data supporting these contentions, and the future directions of this field.

SEARCH STRATEGY

The authors searched the English-language literature for studies published from 2017 to search date (February 15, 2019), using subject headings and keywords to capture the concepts of hyperuricemia and cardiovascular disease in the following databases: MEDLINE (PubMed), Scopus (Elsevier), and Cochrane Library (Wiley). Filters were applied to restrict results to randomized controlled trials (RCTs) or systematic reviews. A separate search was conducted in the same databases to capture the concepts of hypouricemia and cardiovascular disease with no study design restrictions. Search details are available from the authors.

BACKGROUND

Although first recognized by Egyptians in 2640 BC, the history of gout reads like a who's who of medicine, starting with Hippocrates, who, in the fifth century BC, described it as a disease that prevents walking and made several other seminal observations, including that eunuchs do not get gout nor do children or premenopausal women and that it afflicts the rich disproportionately. Galen described tophi and familial predisposition and Anton van Leeuwenhoek (1632–1723) described urate crystals in tophi without knowing their chemical composition. Sydenham gave a brilliant description of an attack of podagra that he himself experienced. Alfred Baring Garrod started the modern era of the study of gout by creating the thread test, which crystalized sodium urate from the serum or urine of patients with gout (the first clinical chemistry test), and suggested the disease could be reduced by decreasing purine-rich foods in the diet, thus implicating hyperuricemia as the pathophysiologic etiology of the disease. Lastly, Joshep Lee Hollander and Daniel J. McCarty demonstrated crystals of sodium urate with polarized microscopy in synovial fluid from patients with acute gouty arthritis.[1]

THE URATE HYPOTHESIS

Based on this convincing set of observations, gout was linked to sodium urate crystals, which are present in soft tissue as tophi and in synovial fluid during a gout attack, which in turn are a consequence of hyperuricemia. To fulfill Koch's postulates, lowering serum urate levels to normal levels eliminates both gout attack and tophi. The synthesis of allopurinol (a xanthine oxidase inhibitor) by George Hitchings and Gertrude Elion resulted in the Nobel Prize in Physiology or in 1988. Thus, in the modern era, the need to treat gout and hyperuricemia by lowering serum urate levels is well accepted and, if done correctly, effectively cures the disease. This paradigm has been extended to treat uric acid nephrolithiasis, tumor lysis syndrome, and, despite some controversy, asymptomatic hyperuricemia if the serum urate levels are very high (>13 mg/dL).[2] This problem has taken on increasing importance as the prevalence of gout and hyperuricemia in the United States has increased. Gout is now present in 4% of the US population and hyperuricemia in more than 20%.[3] These estimates may be low because recent data suggest asymptomatic hyperuricemia patients have a high prevalence of tophi detected by ultrasound.[4]

RECENT ASSOCIATIONS

Hyperuricemia additionally has been implicated in a variety of other conditions, primarily through epidemiologic analysis of large databases. These include hypertension, chronic renal insufficiency, coronary artery disease, myocardial infarction, atherosclerosis, stroke, heart failure, and all-cause mortality. Possibly related are associations of serum urate levels and preeclampsia,[5,6] atrial fibrillation,[7] and pulmonary hypertension.[8] A vast majority of these associations were made through observational studies. Some were cross-sectional, some cohort,[9,10] some large database, and a small number the result of interventional studies. There has been notable inconsistency of the observational studies, and all of them are heavily confounded by comorbid conditions, such as diabetes, obesity, and lifestyle variables. Overall, the corrected odds ratio of cardiovascular disease in gout patients is approximately 4-fold elevated compared with age-matched and gender-matched individuals uncorrected for comorbid conditions.[11] Whether the use of allopurinol could reduce the risk attributable to gout or hyperuricemia is controversial. A Taiwanese study concluded that there was a time-dependent benefit of allopurinol[12] whereas a Danish study concluded that there was no time-dependent or dose-dependent effect of allopurinol[13]; however, there were significant differences in the ways these studies were conducted.

RATIONALE FOR VASCULAR TOXICITY OF URATE

The rationale for the association of hyperuricemia with the range of vascular disorders is in part the role of hyperuricemia (with or without gout) in the metabolic syndrome composed of obesity, glucose intolerance, hypertension, and hyperlipidemia. Teasing out the independent contribution of hyperuricemia to the known risk of this syndrome for all these vascular complications has been extremely difficult. To add to this controversy, the role of sodium urate in physiology has been hotly debated. Higher primates lack the uricase enzyme because of several mutations that have been evolutionarily conserved, suggesting that sodium urate is an important metabolite in higher primates. The problem of gout and hyperuricemia is solely the province of humans because the other higher primates are primarily vegetarian. One explanation for the role of sodium urate is as an antioxidant in physiologic concentrations extracellularly and an intracellular oxidant.[14] With functional uricase, the uric acid levels in all other animals are negligible and the end product of purine degradation is allantoin, a very soluble metabolite that is excreted by the kidney. A competing rationale for loss of uricase is that sodium urate can substitute for sodium chloride to maintain blood pressure in upright biped hominids, especially in a salt-poor environment.

GOUT AND HYPERURICEMIA

At physiologic pH of 7 and body temperature of 37Co, sodium urate is soluble up to a concentration of 6.8 mg/dL. Concentrations higher than that result in crystal formation that occurs in soft tissue for years before clinical gout occurs. Although hyperuricemia is a necessary condition for clinical gout, many other factors are involved. Thus, only a small number of patients with uric acid in the 7.0-mg/dL to 7.9-mg/dL range develop gout. Overall, 80% of people with hyperuricemia remain free of disease. In the Normative Aging Study, the annual incidence of gout for people with sodium urate levels less than 7.0 mg/dL was 0.1%, 0.5% when uric acid was 7.0 mg/dL to 8.9 mg/dL, and 4.9% when the uric acid level was greater than 9.0 mg/dL[15] (for a total of 22% over 5 years). The higher the concentration of urate, however, the more likely it is that gout develops, such that at levels above 13 mg/dL, gout is virtually assured, supporting the Japanese recommendation to treat asymptomatic hyperuricemia but only when the concentration of urate is above 13 mg/dL.[16] Other factors that play a role include dehydration, alcohol, ketosis, diet, drugs, and renal insufficiency, which is 3 times more likely to develop in patients with a serum urate level greater than 9 mg/dL.[17] Although both gout and hyperuricemia have been implicated in vascular risk, there may be different mechanisms at work. Gout is an inflammatory disease, and the activation of cytokines, primarily interleukin (IL)-1 and IL-6, through the inflammasome has profound implications for the endothelium, whereas asymptomatic hyperuricemia is not inflammatory and the effects on the endothelium are considerably milder but could include endothelial dysfunction,[18–21] leading to platelet aggregation vasoconstriction, vascular smooth muscle proliferation adipocyte stimulation, and activation of the renin-angiotensin system[22] by inhibiting nitric oxide synthesis in the juxtaglomerular apparatus. There is some evidence that lowering uric acid levels improves endothelial dysfunction[23–26] Whether the effects of hyperuricemia and gout are additive or synergistic is unknown. Furthermore, at least 2 of the drugs used to treat gout have been believed to ameliorate vascular disease by mechanisms independent of their effects on gout and hyperuricemia. Specifically, allopurinol and febuxostat may reduce reactive oxygen species and free radicals by inhibiting xanthine oxidase independent of the ability to reduce uric acid concentrations,[27] and colchicine may inhibit inflammasome formation systemically, not only in response to uric acid crystals.

OBSERVATIONAL STUDIES

There is substantial epidemiologic evidence that links hyperuricemia to hypertension, including postpartum hypertension[28]; however, for the most part, it is observational and heavily confounded by comorbid conditions, such as obesity, hyperlipidemia, and diabetes. Hyperuricemia is associated with every risk factor for coronary artery disease, including hypertension,[29] atherosclerosis, microalbuminuria, obesity, hypertriglyceridemia, low high-density lipoprotein, hyperinsulinemia, peripheral and carotid artery disease, endothelial dysfunction, renin levels, endothelin level, and C-reactive protein. The sole exception is smoking. Hypertension does have a pathophysiologic rationale because hyperuricemia activates the renin-angiotensin system.[30] These observational studies are summarized in several meta-analyses directed at the association with hypertension,[31] hypertensive retinopathy,[32] coronary artery disease,[33,34] stroke,[35] cardiovascular and all-cause mortality,[36] and chronic renal disease.[37] In studies looking the association of gout with these outcomes, including all-cause mortality, similar findings occur.[38,39] The interventional studies that address this issue are discussed later.

For similar reasons, association of vascular disease (which includes coronary artery disease, atherosclerotic disease, congestive heart failure,[40,41] acute myocardial infarction, stroke, and peripheral vascular disease) and hyperuricemia is controversial because the studies frequently are conflicting. A good example of this is the difference between the National Health and Nutrition Examination Survey I, which followed 5421 patients from 1971 to 1987 and found an association of hyperuricemia with coronary artery disease and all-cause mortality in women (but not men) independent of diastolic blood pressure, obesity, and the use of diuretics and antihypertensives,[42] and the Framingham Heart Study, which followed a total of 6763 patients for 117,376 person-years and found no association between hyperuricemia and cardiovascular risk in either men or women, which does not support the association as an independent risk factor[43] nor by correcting for genetic variation using mendelian randomization,[44] which is less subject to confounding. This study documented the association between hyperuricemia and ischemic heart disease but, using genetic markers to randomize the population, the association was found confounded by body mass index. Observational studies on uricosuric drugs, such as probenecid, for their effect on cardiovascular events, are uncommon and, because they rarely are prescribed, data likely are not forthcoming.[45]

INTERVENTIONAL STUDIES

Interventional trials of urate-lowering therapy for vascular disease prevention are much less common than observational studies. Even rarer are studies to assess the effect of anti-inflammatory drugs used to treat gout on vascular disease prevention. Some interesting data, however, do exist.

URATE-LOWERING THERAPY AND HYPERTENSION

A surprisingly high prevalence of hyperuricemia (up to 10%) is seen in a US populations.[46] Furthermore, there is an observation that 90% of newly diagnosed adolescent hypertensives are hyperuricemic.[47] In addition there is a well-done small trial of allopurinol (200 mg twice a day) in obese adolescent boys with new-onset hypertension, which showed improvement in blood pressure control[48,49] and glomerular filtration rate[50]; however, extending this finding to adults was unsuccessful using allopurinol[51,52] or probenecid[53] despite positive results from observational studies.[54,55] Allopurinol did decrease blood pressure in a trial of hypertensive patients with baseline hyperuricemia,[56] but a Cochrane review concluded that RCT data were insufficient to know whether uric acid–lowering therapy with either allopurinol or febuxostat results in lower blood pressure.[57,58] Some antihypertensive medications may contribute to hyperuricemia by raising serum urate levels, including thiazide diuretics, furosemide, and β-blockers.[59] The relationship between serum urate and hypertension may be mediated by sodium, suggesting that some hyperuricemic patients may have sodium-sensitive hypertension.[60]

CONGESTIVE HEART FAILURE

Allopurinol was unsuccessful in improving chronic heart failure (although there was a trend toward improvement in some subgroups)[61–63] but did improve endothelial function[64] and left ventricular mass,[65] reduced risk of ventricular arrhythmias,[66] and improved exercise tolerance in patients with stable angina.[67,68] Hyperuricemia remains a strong prognostic indicator of poor prognosis in heart failure.[69]

RENAL FUNCTION

Both allopurinol and febuxostat improved glomerular filtration rate albeit by a very small increment in a meta-analysis of RCTs,[70] but this was not seen in a more recent RCT of gout patients.[71] Observational studies suggest a reduction in cardiorenal events in patients treated with xanthine oxidase inhibitors, but this is unproved in clinical trials.[72,73]

CARDIOVASCULAR DISEASE AND ALL-CAUSE MORTALITY

Allopurinol was clearly associated with a reduction in gout in an RCT that failed to show reduction in cardiovascular parameters including hypertension, coronary artery disease, ischemic stroke, heart failure, or renal insufficiency.[74] A propensity-matched observational study found no effect of allopurinol on all-cause mortality.[75] Also, a meta-analysis of RCTs showed no improvement in all-cause mortality[76] but a different meta-analysis suggested allopurinol and oxypurinol reduced cardiovascular events but only at allopurinol doses 300 mg a day or less.[77] A major current controversy is whether there is increased mortality attributable to febuxostat based on data from the Cardiovascular Safety of Febuxostat and Allopurinol in Patients with Gout and Cardiovascular Morbidities (CARES) trial, which showed all-cause mortality was higher in the febuxostat arm even though new cardiovascular events were equivalent. There were many problems with this trial, including high dropout rate, unequal use of nonsteroidal anti-inflammatory agents, many events occurring after the trial ended, and no control group.[78] Lastly, a large cohort study showed no difference in mortality between allopurinol-treated and febuxostat-treated patients[79] in contradiction to the results of the hotly debated CARES trial.[80]

Cerebrovascular disease is even more problematic because some data suggest uric acid elevating therapy improves stroke outcome[81] and some data suggest elevated uric acid worsens outcome.[82]

NONPHARMACEUTICAL INTERVENTIONS

There is no evidence that nonpharmacologic approaches to hyperuricemia, such as diets that restrict purines or dietary purines,[83] Dietary Approaches to Stop Hypertension diet,[84,85] cherry juice,[86] caffeine,[87] vitamin C,[88] and low-fat dairy products,[89] can reduce vascular disease because of their effect to lower hyperuricemia.

SAFETY ISSUES WITH PHARMACOLOGIC INTERVENTIONS

Seven different RCTs of urate-lowering therapy with different mechanisms of action (uricosuric: lesinurad; xanthine oxidase inhibitor: febuxostat; and uricase-pegloticase) all failed to show improved mortality and each had significant safety concerns.[90] For example, in the pegloticase trials, almost all the deaths were in the treatment arm, hypothesized to be a consequence of the H_2O_2-induced oxidation stress that uricase generates when catabolizing urate to allantoin.[91] Febuxostat seems to have higher mortality than allopurinol but not necessarily than no therapy,[92] although there is considerable argument about this conclusion.[93]

ANTI-INFLAMMATORY INTERVENTIONS TO REDUCE VASCULAR EVENTS

There are 2 reports that suggest a preventative effect of treatment of gout on vascular disease that do not reduce uric acid levels. A meta-analysis of RCTs of colchicine suggested a preventive effect,[94] including cerebrovascular disease,[95] and a very large study of canakinumab (an IL-1 antagonist that can be used to treat gout) that reported a small but significant decrease in cardiac events[96] but a definite reduction in gout attacks[97] without a reduction in serum urate levels.

HYPOURICEMIA

Even more recently, there have been observations from both observational and interventional studies that suggest very low levels of serum urate may be associated with adverse outcomes as might be expected from uric acid's role as an antioxidant, especially in the central nervous system. Very low levels of sodium urate are associated with neurodegenerative diseases, such as dementia[98] and Parkinson disease.[99] Some investigators have hypothesized a U-shaped curve for serum urate levels based on data from Taiwan[100,101] and the United States,[102] especially in patients with renal insufficiency.[103] The U-shaped curve describes increased mortality associated with very low levels and very high levels of sodium urate.

SUMMARY

There is an abundance of circumstantial evidence associating hyperuricemia and gout with atherosclerosis; however, much of it is confounded by associated comorbidity. The rationale for vascular injury from gout through inflammation seems a stronger argument than that for hyperuricemia, but neither is conclusively proved to be either true or false. The reason higher primates have lost the enzyme uricase (through germline mutation) remains a mystery but reasons put forth include uric acid as an antioxidant and the possible role of sodium urate as a substitute for sodium chloride in salt-poor environments, but neither of these directly implicates the possibility that gout or hyperuricemia is a risk factor for atherosclerosis. Overall, the interventional data on both canakinumab and colchicine are a stronger argument for gout as a risk factor for vascular disease than hyperuricemia but there are some interventional data implicating hyperuricemia as a risk factor for hypertension that might be an indirect mechanism to link hyperuricemia to atherosclerosis. Future studies are likely to address these questions definitively through large placebo-controlled trials.

REFERENCES

1. Nuki G, Simkin PA. A concise history of gout and hyperuricemia and their treatment. Arthritis Res Ther 2006;8(Suppl 1):S1.
2. Paul BJ, Anoopkumar k, Krishnan V. Asymptomatic hyperuricemia: is it time to intervene. Clin Rheumatol 2017;36:2637–44.
3. Zhu Y, Pandya BJ, Choi HK. prevalence of gout and hyperuricemia in the us general population: the national health and nutrition examination survey 2007-2008. Arthritis Rheum 2011;63:3136–41.
4. Stewart S, Maxwell H, Dalbeth N. Prevalence and discrimination of OMERACT-defined elementary ultrasound lesions of gout in people with asymptomatic hyperuricemia: a Systematic Review and Meta-Analysis. Semin Arthritis Rheum 2019. [Epub ahead of print].
5. Thangaratinam s, Ismail KM, Sharp S, et al. Accuracy of Serum Uric Acid in predicting complications of pre-eclampsia: a systematic review. BJOG 2006;113: 369–78.
6. Koopmans CM, van Pampus MG, Groen H, et al. Accuracy of Serum Uric Acid as a predictive test for maternal complications in pre-eclampsia: bivariate meta-analysis and decision analysis. Eur J Obstet Gynecol Reprod Biol 2009; 146:8–14.
7. Tamariz L, Hernandez F, Bush A, et al. Association between serum uric acid and atrial fibrillation: a systematic review and meta-analysis. Heart Rhythm 2014;11: 1102–8.
8. Kang TU, Park KY, Kim HJ, et al. Association of hyperuricemia and pulmonary hypertension: a systematic review and meta-analysis. Mod Rheumatol 2018; 18:1–28.

9. Bove M, Cicero AFG, Borghi C. the effect of xanthine oxidase inhibitors on blood pressure and renal function. Curr Hypertens Rep 2017;19:95–101.
10. Richette P, Latourte A, Bardin T. Cardiac and renal protective effects of urate lowering therapy. Rheumatology (Oxford) 2018;57(suppl_1):i47–50.
11. Disveld IJM, Fransen J, Rongen GA, et al. Crystal-Proven Gout and Characteristic Gout severity factors are associated with cardiovascular disease. J Rheumatol 2018;45:858–63.
12. Lin HC, Daimon M, Wang CH, et al. Allopurinol, benzbromarone and the risk of coronary heart disease in gout patients: a population-based study. Int J Cardiol 2017;213:85–90.
13. Soltoft Larsen K, Pottegard A, Lindegaard HM, et al. Impact of Urate level on cardiovascular risk in allopurinol treated patients: a nested case-control study. PLoS One 2016;11:e0146172.
14. Gustafsson D, Unwin R. The Pathophysiology of Hyperuricaemia and its possible relationship to cardiovascular disease, morbidity and mortality. BMC Nephrol 2014;14:164.
15. Campion EW, Glynn RJ, Delabry LO. Asymptomatic hyperuricemia:risks and consequences in the normative aging study. Am J Med 1987;82:421–6.
16. Richette P, Latourte A, Bardin T. Cardiac and renal protective effects of urate-lowering therapy. Rheumatology 2018;57(suppl 1):2147–50.
17. Obermayr R, Temmi C, Gutjahr G, et al. Elevated uric acid increases the risk for kidney disease. J Am Soc Nephrol 2008;19:2407–13.
18. George J, Carr E, Davies J, et al. High dose allopurinol improves endothelial function by profoundly reducing vascular oxidative stress and not by lowering uric acid. Circulation 2006;114:2508–16.
19. Kanbay M, Huddam B, Azak A, et al. A Randomized Study of Allopurinol on endothelial function and estimated glomerular filtration rate in asymptomatic hyperuricemic subjects with normal renal function. Clin J Am Soc Nephrol 2011;6: 1887–94.
20. Melendez-Ramirez G, Perez-Mendez O, Lopez-Osorio C, et al. Effect of the treatment with allopurinol on the endothelial function in patients with hyperuricemia. Endocr Res 2012;37:1–6.
21. Doehner W, Schoene N, Rauchhaus M, et al. Effects of xanthine oxidase inhibition with allopurinol on endothelial function and peripheral blood flow in hyperuricemic patients with chronic heart failure: results from two placebo-controlled studies. Circulation 2002;105:2619–24.
22. Corry DB, Eslami P, Yamamoto K, et al. Uric acid causes vascular smooth muscle proliferation and oxidative stress via the vascular renin-angiotensin system. J Hypertens 2008;26:269–75.
23. Alem M. Allopurinol and endothelial function: a systematic review with meta-analysis of randomized controlled trials. Cardiovasc Ther 2018;36:e12432.
24. Cicero AFG, Pirro M, Watts GF, et al. Effect of allopurinol on endothelial function: a systematic review and meta-analysis of randomized placebo-controlled trials. Drugs 2018;78:99–109.
25. Alem MM, Alshehri AM, Cahusac PM, et al. Effect of xanthine oxidase inhibition on arterial stiffness in patients with chronic heart failure. Clin Med Insights Cardiol 2018;12. 1179546818779584.
26. Alshahawry M, Shahin SM, Elsaid TW, et al. Effect of febuxostat on the endothelial dysfunction in hemodialysis patients: a randomized placebo-controlled double-blind study. Am J Nephrol 2017;45:452–8.

27. Das DK, Engelman RM, Clement R, et al. Role of xanthine oxidase inhibitor as free radical scavender: a novel mechanism of action of allopurinol and oxypurinol in myocardial salvage. Biochem Biophys Res Commun 1987;148:314–9.
28. Marrs CC, Rahman M, Dixon L, et al. The association of Hyperuricemia and Immediate Postpartum hypertension in Women without a diagnosis of Chronic Hypertension. Hypertens Pregnancy 2018;37:126–30.
29. Grayson PC, Kim SY, LaValley M, et al. hyperuricemia and incident hypertension: a systematic review and meta-analysis. Arthritis Care Res 2011;63:102–10.
30. Larsen KS, Pottegard A, Lindegaard HM, et al. Effect of allopurinol on cardiovascular outcomesin hyperuricemic patients: a cohort study. Am J Med 2016; 129:299–306.
31. Wang J, Qin T, Li Y, et al. Hyperuricemia and the risk of incident hypertension: a systematic review and meta-analysis of observational studies. PLoS One 2014; 9:0114259.
32. Chen X, Meng Y, Li J, et al. Serum uric acid concentration is associated with hypertensive retinopathy in hyperuricemic chinese adults. BMC Ophthalmol 2017; 17:83.
33. Kim S, Guevara J, Kim K, et al. Hyperuricemia and coronary artery disease: a systematic review and meta-analysis. Arthritis Care Res 2010;62:170–80.
34. Li M, Hu X, Fan Y, et al. Hyperuricemia and the risk for coronary heart disease morbidity and mortality: a systematic review and dose-response meta-analysis. Sci Rep 2016;6:19520.
35. Kim S, Guervara J, Kim K, et al. Hyperuricemia and the risk of Stroke: a systematic review and meta-analysis. Arthritis Care Res 2009;61:885–92.
36. Zhao G, Huang L, Song M, et al. Baseline serum uric acid level as a predictor of cardiovascular disease related mortality and all-cause mortality: a meta-analysis of prospective studies. Atherosclerosis 2013;231:61–8.
37. Li L, Yang C, Zhao Y, et al. Is hyperuricemia an independent risk factor for new-onset chronic kidney disease? A systematic review and meta-analysis based on observational cohort studies. BMC Nephrol 2014;15:122.
38. Lottmann k, Chen X, Schadlich PK. Association between Gout and All-Cause as well as cardiovascular mortality: a systematic review. Curr Rheumatol Rep 2012; 14:195–202.
39. Clarson LE, Chadratre P, Hider SL, et al. Increased Cardiovascular Mortality Associated with Gout: a systematic review and meta-analysis. Eur J Prev Cardiol 2015;22:335–43.
40. Tamariz L, Harzand A, Palacio A, et al. Uric acid as a predictor of all-cause mortality in heart failure: a meta-analysis. Congest Heart Fail 2011;17:25–30.
41. Huang H, Huang B, Li Y, et al. Uric acid and the risk of heart failure: asystematic review and meta-analysis. Eur J Heart Fail 2014;16:15–24.
42. Reedman DS, Williamson DF, Gunter EW, et al. Relationof serum uric acid to mortality and ischemic heart disease: the NHANES 1 Epidemiologic Followup Study. Am J Epidemiol 1995;141:637–44.
43. Culleton BF, Larson MB, Kannel WB, et al. Serum uric acid and risk for cardiovascular disease and death. Ann Intern Med 1999;131:7–13.
44. Kleber M, Delgado G, Grammer TB, et al. Uric Acid and Cardiovascular Events: A Mendelian Randomization Study. J AM Soc Nephrol 2015;26:2831–8.
45. Kim SC, Neogi T, Kang EH. Cardiovascular risks of probenecid versus allopurinol in older patients with gout. J Am Coll Cardiol 2018;71:994–1004.
46. Li N, Zhang S, Li W, et al. Prevalence of Hyperuricemia and its related risk factors among preschool children from China. Sci Rep 2017;7:9448.

47. Feig DI, Johnson RJ. Hyperuricemia in childhood primary hypertension. Hypertension 2003;42:247–52.
48. Feig DI, Soletsky B, Johnson RJ. Effect of Allopurinol on blood pressure of adolescents with newly diagnosed essential hypertension. JAMA 2008;300: 924–32.
49. Soletsky B, Feig DI. Uric acid reduction rectifies prehypertension in obese adolescents. Hypertension 2012;60:1148–56.
50. Ghane Sharbof F, Assadi F. Effect of allopurinol on the glomerular filtration rate of children with chronic kidney disease. Pediatr Nephrol 2018;33:1405–9.
51. Beattie CJ, Fulton RL, Higgins P. Allopurinol initiation and change in blood pressure in older adults with hypertension. Hypertension 2014;64:1102–7.
52. Segal M, Srinivas T, Mohandas R, et al. The effect of the addition of allopurinol on blood pressure control in African Americans Treated with a thiazide-like diuretic. J Am Soc Hypertens 2015;9:610–9.
53. McMullan CJ, Borgi L, Fisher N, et al. Effect of urate lowering on renin-angiotensin –system activation and ambulatory Blood Pressure: a randomized controlled trial. Clin J Am Soc Nephrol 2017;12:807–16.
54. Beattie CJ, Fulton RL, Higgins P, et al. Allopurinol Initiation and change in blood pressure in older adults with hypertension. Hypertension 2014;64:1102–7.
55. Agarwal V, Hans N, Messerli FH. Effect of allopurinol on blood pressure: a systematic review and meta-analysis. J Clin Hypertens 2013;15:435–42.
56. Kanbay M, Ozkara A, Selcoki Y, et al. Effect of treatment of hyperuricemia with allopurinol on blood pressure, creatinine clearance, and proteinuria in patients with normal renal functions. Int Urol Nephrol 2007;39:1227–33.
57. Gois PHF, Souza ERM. Pharmacotherapy for hyperuricemia in hypertensive patients. Cochrane Database Syst Rev 2017;(4):CD008652.
58. Gunawardhana L, McLean L, Punzi HA, et al. Effect of febuxostat on ambulatory blood pressure in subjects with hyperuricemia and hypertrension: a phase 2 randomized placebo-controlled study. J Am Heart Assoc 2017;6(11) [pii: e006683].
59. Juraschek Metoprolol increases uric acid and risk of gout in African Americans with Chronic Kidney Diseasetributed to Hypertension. Am J Hypertens 2017;30: 871–5.
60. Todd AS, Walker RJ, MacGinley RJ, et al. Dietary sodium modifies serum uric acid concentration in humans. Am J Hypertens 2017;30:1196–202.
61. Givertz M, Anstrom K, Redfield M, et al. Effects of xanthine oxidase inhibition in hyperuricemic heart failure patients. The xanthine oxidase inhibition for hyperuricemic heart failure patients (EXACT-HF) study. Circulation 2015;131:1763–71.
62. Hare JM, Mangal B, Brown J, et al. Impact of oxypurinol in patients with symptomatic heart failure. J Am Coll Cardiol 2008;51:2301–9.
63. Wei L, Mackenzie IS, Chen Y, et al. Impact of Allopurinol use on Urate concentration and cardiovascular outcome. Br J Clin Pharmacol 2011;71:600–7.
64. Kanbay M, Siriopol D, Nistor I, Elcicoglu OC, et al. Effects of allopurinol on endothelial dysfunction: a meta-analysis. Am J Nephrol 2014;39:348–56.
65. Engberding N, Spiekermann S, Schaefer A, et al. Allopurinol attenuates left ventricular remodeling and dysfunction after experimental myocardial infarction: a new action for an old drug. Circulation 2004;110:2175–9.
66. Singh JA, Cleveland J. Allopurinol and the risk of ventricular arrhythmias in the elderly: A study using US Medicare Data. BMC Med 2017;15:59.

67. Norman A, Ang D, Ogston S, et al. Effect of high dose allopurinol on exercise in patients with stable angina: a randomized, placebo controlled crossover trial. Lancet 2010;375:2161–7.
68. Okafor ON, Farrington K, Gorog DA. Allopurinol as a therapeutic option in Cardiovascular Disease. Pharmacol Ther 2017;172:139–50.
69. Mantovani A, Targher G, Temporelli PL, et al. Prognostic Impact of elevated serum uric acid on long-term outcome in patients with chronic heart failure: a post hoc analysis of the GISSI-HF trial. Metabolism 2018;83:205–15.
70. Kanji T, Ganghi M, Chase C, et al. Urate lowering therapy to improverenal outcomes in patients with chronic kidney disease: systematic review and meta-analysis. BMC Nephrol 2015;16:58.
71. Saag K, Whelton A, Becker MA, et al. Impact of Febuxostat in gout patients with moderate-to-severe renal impairment. Arthritis Rheum 2016;68:2035–40.
72. Srivastava A, Kaze AD, McMullan CJ, et al. Uric Acid and the risks of kidney failure and Death in Individuals with CKD. Am J Kidney Dis 2018;71:362–70.
73. Su X, Xu B, Yan B, et al. Effect of uric acid-lowering therapy in patients with chronic kidney disease: a meta-analysis. PLoS One 2017;12:e0187550.
74. Keenan T, Zhao W, Rasheed A, et al. Causal Assessment of serum urate levels in cardiovascular diseases through a Mendelian Randomization Study Jour. Am Coll Card 2016;67:407–16.
75. Kuo C-F, Grainge MJ, Mallen C, et al. Effect of allopurinol on all-cause mortality in adults with incident gout: propensity-matched landmark analysis. Rheumatology 2015;54:2145–50.
76. Zhang T, Pope JE. Cardiovascular effects of Urate-lowering therapies in patients with chronic gout: a systematic review and meta-analysis. Rheumatology 2017; 56:1144–53.
77. Bredemeier M, Lopes LM, Eisenreich MA, et al. Xanthine oxidase inhibitors for the prevention of cardiovascular events: a systematic review and meta-analysis of randomized controlled trials. BMC Cardiovasc Disord 2018;18: 24–35.
78. White WB, Saag KG, Becker MA, et al. Cardiovascular safety of febuxostat or allopurinol in patients with gout. N Engl J Med 2018;378:1200–10.
79. Zhang M, Solomon DH, Desai RJ, et al. Assessment of Cardiovascular risk in older patients with gout initiating febuxostat versus Allopurinol: a Population based study. Circulation 2018;138:1116–26.
80. Choi H, Neogi T, Stamp L, et al. New perspectives in rheumatology: implications of the cardiovascular safety of febuxostat and allopurinol in patients with gout and cardiovascular disease. Arthritis Rheumatol 2018;70:1702–9.
81. Chamorro A, Amaro S, Castellanos M, et al. Uric acid therapy improves the outcomes of stroke patients treated with intravenous plasminogen activator and mechanical thrombectomy. Int J Stroke 2017;12:377–82.
82. Du L, Ma J, Zhang X. Higher serum uric acid may contribute to cerebral infarction in patients with type 2 Diabetes Mellitus: a meta-analysis. J Mol Neurosci 2017;61:25–31.
83. Richette P, Doherty M, Pascual E, et al. 2016 updated EULAR evidence=-based recommendations for the management of gout. Ann Rheum Dis 2017;78:29–42.
84. Juraschek SP, White K, Tang O, et al. Effect of a dietary approach to stop hypertension (DASH) Diet Intervention on Serum Uric Acid in African Americans with Hypertension. Arthritis Care Res 2018;70:1509–16.
85. Tang O, Miller ER 3rd, Gelber AC, et al. DASH diet and change in serum uric acid over time. Clin Rheumatol 2017;36:1413–7.

86. Zhang Y, Neogi T, Chen C. Cherry Consumption and the risk of recurrent gout attacks. Arthritis Rheum 2012;64:4004–11.
87. Park KY, Kim HJ, Ahn HS. Effects of Coffee Consumption on serum uric acid: systematic review and meta-analysis. Semin Arthritis Rheum 2016;45:580–6.
88. Juraschek SP, Miller ER, Gelber AC. Effect of oral Vitamin C supplementation on serum uric acid: a meta-analysis of randomized controlled trials. Arthritis Care Res 2011;63:1295–306.
89. Dalbeth N, Palmano K. Effects of dairy intake on hyperuricemia and gout. Curr Rheumatol Rep 2011;13:132–7.
90. Perez-Gomez MV, Bartsch L-A, Castillo-Rodriquez E, et al. Potential dangers of serum urate-lowering therapy. Am J Med 2019;132(4):457–67.
91. Becker MA, Baraf HS, Yood RA, et al. Long-term safety of pegloticase in chronic gout refractory to conventional treatment. Ann Rheum Dis 2013;72:1469–74.
92. Zhang M, Solomon DH, Desai RJ, et al. Assessment of cardiovascular risk in older patients with gout initiating febuxostat versus allopurinol: a population-based cohort study. Circulation 2019;132(4):457–67.
93. Kim SC, Schneeweiss S, Choudry N, et al. Effects of xanthine oxidase inhibitors on cardiovascular disease in patients with gout: a cohort study. Am J Med 2015;128:653.e7-16.
94. Verma S, Elkelboom JW, Nidorf SM, et al. Colchicine in cardiac disease: a systematic review and meta-analysis of randomized controlled trials. BMC Cardiovasc Disord 2015;15:96–111.
95. Tsivgoulis G, Katsanos AH, Giannopoulos G, et al. The role of colchicine in the prevention of cerebrovascular ischemia. Curr Pharm Des 2018;24:668–74.
96. Ridker PM, Everett BM, Thuren T, et al, for the CANTOS Trial Group. Antiinflammatory therapy canakinumab atherosclerotic disease. N Engl J Med 2017;377:1119–31.
97. Solomon DH, Glynn RJ, MacFadyen JG, et al. Relationship of Interleukin 1Beta Blockade with Incident gout and serum uric acid levels: exploratory analysis of a randomized controlled trial. Ann Intern Med 2018;169:535–42.
98. Euser SM, Hofman A, Westendorp RG, et al. Serum uric acid and cognitive function and dementia. Brain 2009;132:377–82.
99. Ascherio A, LeWitt PA, Xu K, et al. Urate as a predictor of the rate of clinical decline in Parkinson Disease. Arch Neurol 2009;66:1460–8.
100. Tseng WC, Chen YT, Ou SM, et al. U-shaped association between serum uric acid levels with cardiovascular and all-cause mortality in the elderly: the role of malnourishment. J Am Heart Assoc 2018;7:4.
101. Yang Y, Zhang Y, Li Y, et al. U shaped relationship between functional outcome and serum uric acid in ischemic stroke. Cell Physiol Biochem 2018;47:2369–79.
102. Kobylecki CJ, Afzal S, Nordestgaard BG. Plasma urate, cancer incidence, and all-cause mortality: a mendelian randomization study. Clin Chem 2017;63:1151–60.
103. Odden MC, Amadu AR, Smit E, et al. Uric acid levels, kidney function, and cardiovascular mortality in US adults: National Health and Nutrition Examination Survey (NHANES) 1988-1994 and 1999-2002. Am J Kidney Dis 2014;64:550–7.

Are There Benefits and Risks to Biosimilars from a Patient Perspective?

Jonathan Kay, MD

KEYWORDS

- Biosimilar pharmaceuticals • Tumor necrosis factor antagonists & inhibitors
- Infliximab • Switching • Drug costs • Rheumatic diseases

KEY POINTS

- A biosimilar that has been approved by a regulatory authority in a highly regulated area is like another batch of its reference product but produced by a different manufacturer.
- A patient should derive the same therapeutic benefit from a biosimilar as from its reference product.
- A patient treated with a reference product can change to its approved biosimilar without loss of efficacy or an increase in safety risk.
- A biosimilar should cost significantly less than its reference product and at least a portion of the cost savings realized from using a biosimilar should be passed on to the patient.

Biologic medications provide very effective treatment of rheumatologic diseases, but their high cost often limits their availability to patients. To increase access to these therapies, once a biologic medication no longer is protected by patent, biosimilars have been developed as copies of the bio-originator (reference product) that are intended to be marketed at prices lower than that of the reference product. On March 23, 2010, President Barack Obama signed the Affordable Care Act into law. Section 7002 of this Act (also known as the Biologics Price Competition and Innovation [BPCI] Act of 2009) established an abbreviated pathway for the review and approval of biosimilars by the United States Food and Drug Administration (FDA).[1] In this legislation, a biosimilar is defined as being "highly similar to the reference product notwithstanding minor differences in clinically inactive components," and that "there are no clinically meaningful differences between the biologic product and the reference

Disclosure Statement: Research Support (paid to the University of Massachusetts Medical School): Pfizer.; UCB, Inc. Consultant: AbbVie Inc.; Boehringer Ingelheim GmbH; Celltrion Healthcare Co. Ltd.; Merck Sharp & Dohme Corp.; Pfizer Inc; Samsung Bioepis; Sandoz Inc; UCB, Inc.
Rheumatology Center, Memorial Campus, UMass Memorial Medical Center and University of Massachusetts Medical School, 119 Belmont Street, Worcester, MA 01605, USA
E-mail address: jonathan.kay@umassmemorial.org

Rheum Dis Clin N Am 45 (2019) 465–476
https://doi.org/10.1016/j.rdc.2019.04.001 rheumatic.theclinics.com

product in terms of the safety, purity, and potency of the product." To fulfill this definition, a biosimilar candidate must undergo rigorous analytical and clinical assessment, in comparison with its reference product.

Because a biosimilar must have equivalent pharmacokinetic parameters and efficacy and comparable safety and immunogenicity with its reference product, the only significant difference between the two should be cost. The biosimilar should provide patients with essentially the same medication as its reference product, but at a lower price. From a patient's perspective, the benefit of a lower-cost biosimilar that has been approved by a regulatory authority in a highly regulated area should be its therapeutic effect with a reduced financial burden.

As of April 2019, 19 biosimilars had been approved in the United States, offering the potential for meaningful cost savings when treating chronic diseases that require long-term use of expensive biologic medications.[2] Of the 19 FDA-approved biosimilars, 1 is a rituximab biosimilar approved for the treatment of non-Hodgkin lymphoma and 8 are tumor necrosis factor inhibitors approved for the treatment of rheumatoid arthritis, psoriatic arthritis, and axial spondyloarthritis, among other indications: 3 adalimumab biosimilars, 2 etanercept biosimilars, and 3 infliximab biosimilars. However, only 2 of the 3 infliximab biosimilars (Inflectra [infliximab-dyyb] and Renflexis [infliximab-abda]) are currently marketed in the United States. Because of patent-related issues, the adalimumab, etanercept, and rituximab biosimilars are not yet available.

A BIOSIMILAR IS LIKE ANOTHER BATCH OF ITS REFERENCE PRODUCT

A biosimilar that has been approved by a regulatory authority in a highly regulated area is like another batch of its reference product, but produced by a different manufacturer.[3] To develop a biosimilar, the biosimilar manufacturer purchases available lots of the reference product and performs an extensive array of analytical studies to characterize its structure and function. Based on this information, the biosimilar manufacturer sets out to replicate the reference product[4] (**Fig. 1**). However, because the biosimilar manufacturer does not have access to the proprietary information that is held by the manufacturer of the reference product, the biosimilar will be a close, but not exact, reproduction of the reference product.

Having determined the primary structure of the reference product, the biosimilar manufacturer synthesizes a gene that encodes this amino acid sequence. However, because there are redundant codons for 18 of the 20 amino acids, the nucleotide sequence for the biosimilar may not be identical to that of the gene for the reference product. Regardless, the gene synthesized to produce the biosimilar must and will encode the same amino acid sequence as that of the reference product. This gene is then inserted into a vector, which may or may not be the same as that used to produce the reference product, and the vector then is used to transfect a cell line in which the biosimilar will be produced.

During the extensive structural analysis of the reference product, the biosimilar manufacturer has characterized its posttranslational modifications. Many of these posttranslational modifications, such as glycosylation and disulfide bond formation, are necessary to achieve the appropriate structure and function of the therapeutic protein. To reproduce these, the biosimilar manufacturer chooses a cell line that is most likely to recapitulate these posttranslational modifications. This cell line often is very closely related to that in which the reference product is produced. However, because the identity of the cell line in which the reference product is manufactured is proprietary, the cell line used for production of the biosimilar may not be the same as that used for the reference product.

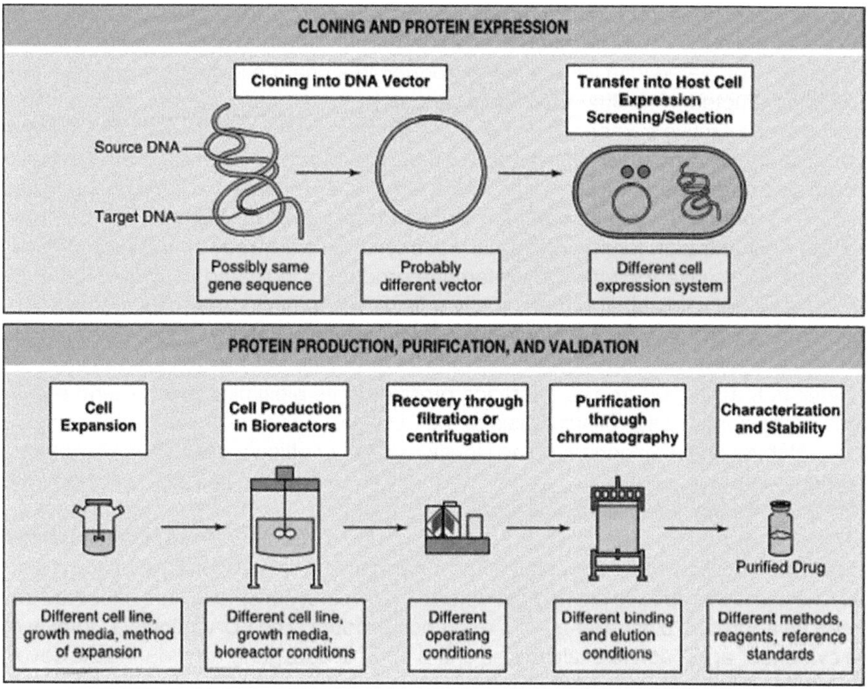

Fig. 1. Manufacturing process for biosimilars. (*From* Mellstedt H, Niederwieser D, Ludwig H. The challenge of biosimilars. Ann Oncol 2008;19(3):411–19; with permission.)

After the cell line has been transfected with the gene encoding the biosimilar, it is grown in culture. The medium and conditions used to grow the biosimilar cell line may or may not be the same as those used to produce the reference product, since that information is also proprietary. As the cells replicate, the cell culture is expanded by transfer to vessels with larger and larger volumes. Eventually, the cell line is grown in large bioreactors containing thousands of liters of culture medium to yield sufficient quantities of the biosimilar for therapeutic use. These bioreactors are similar, but may not be identical, to those used to grow the reference product cell line.

Once the large-scale cell cultures have produced the therapeutic protein, it is harvested from the medium and concentrated by centrifugation, filtration, or chromatography. The process by which the protein is recovered may differ from that proprietary process by which the reference product is harvested from its cell culture. Once purified, the biosimilar candidate is subjected to a variety of analytical assays to demonstrate that it is "highly similar" to its reference product.

The potential differences between the conditions used to produce the reference product and those used to produce the biosimilar candidate may result in slight differences between the therapeutic proteins. However, these differences must not be "clinically significant," if the biosimilar candidate is to be approved by a regulatory agency in a highly regulated area.

A BIOSIMILAR SHOULD PROVIDE THE SAME THERAPEUTIC BENEFIT AS ITS REFERENCE PRODUCT

An approved biosimilar is highly similar to its reference product in structure and function, "without clinically meaningful differences."[5] Extensive comparative analytical studies have confirmed the structural and functional similarity of the biosimilar candidate to its reference product. The biosimilar candidate must demonstrate similar efficacy and safety, compared with its reference product, in a pharmacokinetic study that typically is conducted in healthy volunteers, and in at least 1 randomized, double-blind, parallel group, active comparator clinical trial conducted in patients with that disease indication which is most sensitive to detect potential differences between the biosimilar candidate and its reference product.[5] If an appropriate biomarker is available to assess response to therapy, such as the absolute neutrophil count for filgrastim or the blood glucose concentration for insulin, a pharmacodynamic study may be performed in patients with a disease for which the reference product is indicated. However, no such biomarker is yet available that adequately reflects response to treatment in rheumatologic diseases. In these clinical studies, the biosimilar candidate must also demonstrate comparable safety and immunogenicity with its reference product.

Patients transitioned from a reference product to its biosimilar in long-term extensions of the comparative clinical trials of the FDA-approved biosimilar tumor necrosis factor inhibitors have experienced no significant loss of efficacy or increase in adverse events or immunogenicity.[6–14] Thus, a patient should derive the same therapeutic benefit from a biosimilar as from its reference product.

The goal of a biosimilar development program is to "reduce residual uncertainty," thereby demonstrating that the biosimilar candidate and reference product are essentially the same therapeutic protein. No differences in safety or efficacy are expected between an approved biosimilar and its reference product. The FDA follows a "totality of the evidence" approach to evaluate the entire body of data generated during the development of a biosimilar candidate.[15] All aspects of the biosimilar development program are considered together and are given equal weight. Once equivalent efficacy and comparable safety of the biosimilar and its reference product have been demonstrated, an approved biosimilar can be considered like another batch of its reference product.

Because efficacy and safety of the reference product already have been demonstrated in each indication for which it has been approved, efficacy of the biosimilar need not be demonstrated in every indication. Data from randomized, placebo-controlled clinical trials and subsequent accumulated clinical experience with the reference product in all indications for which it is approved, but which no longer are protected by patent, can be extrapolated to the biosimilar. This opportunity for "extrapolation of indications" in the abbreviated biosimilar approval pathway markedly reduces development costs by eliminating the need to conduct expensive clinical trials of the biosimilar candidate in each indication for which approval is sought.

A biosimilar may have fewer associated adverse effects and be less immunogenic than its reference product, provided that pharmacokinetic parameters and efficacy are equivalent. For example, when compared in a randomized, double-blind clinical trial, the biosimilar etanercept SB4 (etanercept-yrko) caused fewer injection site reactions and had a lower incidence of antidrug antibodies than reference etanercept.[16] However, most approved biosimilars have demonstrated adverse event profiles and immunogenicity similar to those of their reference products. Thus, a patient should derive the same therapeutic benefit from an approved biosimilar as from its reference product, with comparable safety.

A PATIENT CAN CHANGE FROM A REFERENCE PRODUCT TO ITS APPROVED BIOSIMILAR WITHOUT LOSS OF EFFICACY OR INCREASED SAFETY RISK

A patient treated with a reference product can change to its approved biosimilar without loss of efficacy or increase in safety risk. In partnership with the patient, a health care provider may intentionally alter therapy for economic reasons ("nonmedical changing"), if the cost of a biosimilar is less than that of its reference product. A patient may also be changed to a biosimilar for medical reasons when she or he is not responding adequately to a drug other than the reference product and a lower-cost biosimilar is chosen as an alternative treatment.[17] Although the BPCI Act defines "interchangeability" as when a "biological product may be substituted for the reference product without the intervention of the healthcare provider who prescribed the reference product," no biosimilar has yet sought this regulatory designation that is unique to the United States.

Bio-originators have undergone multiple manufacturing process changes after marketing approval,[18] which have resulted in batch-to-batch variation in molecular characteristics and sometimes in functional properties.[19,20] Lots of a bio-originator sourced in the European Union may differ in some product attributes even from lots of the same drug sourced in the United States.[21] Thus, over time, patients already have been switched unknowingly between variants of the same biopharmaceutical that may differ as much or as little as do biosimilars from their reference products and from one another. The results of the NOR-SWITCH trial and the observations in the Danish DANBIO registry support the practice of changing patients with disease activity that is, controlled on a reference product to treatment with its biosimilar.

NOR-SWITCH is the only prospective, double-blind, randomized controlled trial that has compared transitioning from a reference product with its biosimilar to continued treatment with the reference product.[22] In this study, 482 patients with any of the 6 inflammatory diseases for which infliximab is indicated, and who had exhibited stable disease activity over the previous 6 months, were randomly allocated equally, either to continue treatment with reference infliximab or to change from reference infliximab to biosimilar infliximab CT-P13 (infliximab-dyyb). The primary endpoint was worsening of disease activity up to 52 weeks, as assessed using a different disease-specific index for each of the 6 inflammatory diseases or by agreement between the patient and the investigator that persistent disease activity necessitated a "major change in treatment." This study demonstrated that changing to the biosimilar was noninferior to continuing treatment with the reference product over 52 weeks in the combined population of patients with the 6 inflammatory diseases. Trough drug concentrations throughout the study and the incidence of adverse events, infusion reactions, and antidrug antibodies were similar between the patients who changed to the biosimilar and those who continued treatment with the reference product.

In the DANBIO registry, patients with rheumatoid arthritis, psoriatic arthritis, and axial spondyloarthritis who underwent a government-mandated change from reference infliximab to biosimilar infliximab CT-P13 exhibited similar disease activity before and after undergoing this therapeutic substitution.[23] The crude retention rate after 1 year on biosimilar infliximab was similar to that in a historical cohort of patients treated with reference infliximab; the retention rate adjusted for a variety of baseline variables was only slightly lower for those treated with the biosimilar than for those treated with the reference product.

When a patient with stable disease activity that has been controlled on treatment with a reference product is changed to its biosimilar, he or she may anticipate decreased efficacy and lesser safety of the biosimilar and therefore may experience subjective disease worsening or adverse events on the new medication. This nocebo effect has resulted in decreased acceptance of and lower retention rates on biosimilar infliximab CT-P13 than on treatment with reference infliximab.[24] Collaborative discussion with patients, educating them about the rationale for changing to the biosimilar, reassuring them about the equivalent efficacy and comparable safety of the biosimilar with its reference product, and counseling them about the possible nocebo response may mitigate this and improve acceptance of the biosimilar and hence the clinical outcome.[25]

A BIOSIMILAR SHOULD COST SIGNIFICANTLY LESS THAN ITS REFERENCE PRODUCT

Because an approved biosimilar is like another batch of the reference product, the only difference should be cost. The price at which a biosimilar is sold should be lower than that of its reference product. Otherwise, there would be no benefit of biosimilars to the health care system. However, patients should partake of these cost savings.

In 2006, the European Medicines Agency (EMA) approved Omnitrope, a biosimilar recombinant human growth hormone, as the first biosimilar in the European Union. Over the subsequent 13 years, additional biosimilars have been approved and, as of April 2019, 56 of 60 biosimilars approved by the EMA were commercially available.[26] Market competition in many European Economic Area (EEA) countries has resulted in significant price reductions for biosimilars, compared with their reference products. Such market competition has resulted in lower prices and increased sales volume, not only for the biosimilars but also for other products in the same therapeutic class for which biosimilars are not available.[27]

The greatest cost savings resulting from the introduction of biosimilars have occurred in countries in which there is a single-payer health care system with a competitive bidding process to acquire medications. In Norway, hospital-administered medications are purchased by a government agency through a competitive tender system. Using this process, the single payer has been able to negotiate aggressively for discounted acquisition costs, resulting in savings of up to 70% in Norway for biosimilar infliximab compared with its reference product.[28] Alternatively, competition created by the introduction of a biosimilar may give rise to savings by driving down the price of its reference product. In late October 2018, AbbVie won the Swedish national tender for adalimumab by dropping the price for reference adalimumab by 80%.[29] Thus, in countries with a single national health insurer and a "winner-take-all" competitive bidding process for drug acquisition, the promise of meaningful cost savings is being realized with the availability of biosimilars.[30]

In contrast to the significant price reductions seen with biosimilars in some EEA countries, the first 2 biosimilars marketed in the United States (filgrastim-sndz and infliximab-dyyb) were each launched with a wholesale acquisition cost (WAC) only 15% lower than that of its reference product. Although the second infliximab biosimilar approved in the United States, infliximab-abda, was launched with a WAC 35% lower than that of its reference product and 20% lower than that of infliximab-dyyb, it was more expensive than the infliximab biosimilars marketed in other countries.[31]

In the United States, biopharmaceuticals are often dispensed to patients by specialty pharmacies run by pharmacy benefit managers (PBMs). These PBMs are third-parties that charge a fee to administer prescription drug programs for commercial, government, and self-insured employer plans.[32,33] The PBMs negotiate rebates and discounts with drug manufacturers, based on the list price of a drug: the higher the list price, the larger the discount and rebate that can be negotiated. The PBM typically returns some, but not all, of these cost savings to the plan sponsor. Thus, it is to the advantage of a PBM to place higher-priced drugs, for which it has negotiated significant rebates and discounts, on formulary. The balance of the rebate and discount that is not returned to the plan sponsor contributes to the PBM's profits. For that reason, a biosimilar with a list price lower than that of its reference product may be less attractive to a PBM.

To encourage prescription of a reference product with a list price higher than that of its biosimilar, a PBM may institute a “prior authorization” process that favors the reference product over the biosimilar. Alternatively, a PBM may incentivize patients to use the reference product preferentially by placing it in a lower “tier” than the biosimilar, requiring a lower copayment of the patient for the reference product. There may be a requirement for “step therapy” (also known as “fail first”), whereby a patient must first demonstrate an inadequate response to a lower-priced medication, such as a conventional synthetic disease-modifying antirheumatic drug, before being allowed treatment with a biopharmaceutical. In some instances, a PBM may not authorize treatment with a biosimilar unless a patient has first tried and responded inadequately to treatment with the reference product.[34] In such a situation, treatment with the biosimilar should be contraindicated, because the biosimilar is essentially the same molecule.[35] A PBM even may have a restricted formulary in which the reference product, but not the biosimilar, is available.

In the United States, medications administered in a health care facility are reimbursed by Medicare Part B according to the “Average Sales Price” (ASP) that reflects all types of discounts, such as rebates and volume discounts. Such “physician-administered drugs” are reimbursed at 106% of the ASP.[36] Initially, all biosimilar infliximab products were grouped under the HCPCS code Q5102 and were reimbursed at 106% of the ASP of the reference product. As of April 1, 2018, the Medicare program changed the coding and reimbursement for biosimilar infliximab to allow each product to have its own ASP, replacing the grouped HCPCS code Q5102 with individual HCPCS codes Q5103 for biosimilar infliximab-dyyb and Q5104 for biosimilar infliximab-abda.[37] This introduction of unique HCPCS codes for individual biosimilars created price competition among biosimilars and resulted in further reductions in the cost of infliximab, both of the reference product and of each of the 2 biosimilars[38] (**Fig. 2**). However, unlike the experience in EEA countries, the availability of 2 biosimilar infliximabs in the United States has resulted in only a 17% to 24% reduction of the ASP of biosimilar infliximab, compared with that of its reference product.[38]

Biosimilar infliximab-dyyb was first marketed in the United States on November 28, 2016,[39] with a WAC priced 15% lower than that of reference infliximab.[40] However, the ASP of reference infliximab, which takes into account rebates and volume discounts, was actually $181 per 100 mg (18%) lower than that of the biosimilar. The lower effective price of reference infliximab and the initial hesitancy of health care providers to prescribe a biosimilar in place of its reference product resulted in much lower sales of infliximab-dyyb than of reference infliximab through the end of that year. During the fourth quarter of 2016, infliximab-dyyb sales were only $3.7 million, compared with reference infliximab sales of $1.17 billion.[41] During the first half of 2017, infliximab-dyyb sales still were only $43.7 million, compared with $2.24 billion for the reference product.

The ASPs of infliximab biosimilars in the United States have decreased by nearly 50%, since the launch of infliximab-dyyb.[38] On July 24, 2017, a second infliximab biosimilar, infliximab-abda, was introduced to the market in the United States with a WAC priced 35% lower than that of reference infliximab. However, because Medicare grouped both infliximab biosimilars under a single HCPCS code, the initial ASP for infliximab-abda was the same as that for infliximab-dyyb and was $55 per 100 mg less than that of reference infliximab. When the Medicare program replaced the single HCPCS code for both infliximab biosimilars with individual HCPCS codes for each biosimilar infliximab, in the second quarter of 2018, the ASP for each infliximab biosimilar was about $130 per 100 mg less than that of reference infliximab.[42] However, market competition initiated by the introduction of the second infliximab biosimilar prompted

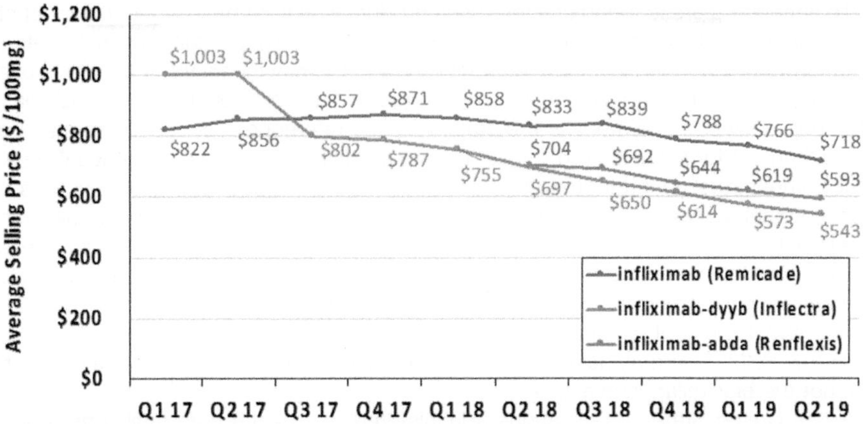

Fig. 2. Average Selling Prices (ASPs) of both reference infliximab and infliximab biosimilars have decreased over time. (*Data from* the Centers for Medicare and Medicaid Services. Medicare Part B Drug Average Sales Price. 2017, 2018, and 2019 ASP Drug Pricing Files. 2019; https://www.cms.gov/Medicare/Medicare-Fee-for-Service-Part-B-Drugs/McrPartBDrug AvgSalesPrice/2019ASPFiles.html. Accessed March 9, 2019.)

further decreases in the ASP of all infliximabs, both reference product and biosimilars. Over the subsequent year, the ASP of reference infliximab decreased by $115 per 100 mg and the ASPs of infliximab-abda and infliximab-dyyb decreased by $111 and $154 per 100 mg, respectively. As of the second quarter of 2019, the ASP of infliximab-dyyb was the lowest, being $50 per 100 mg less than the ASP of infliximab-abda and $175 per 100 mg less than that of reference infliximab.

With the current health care system in the United States, the cost savings realized from using a biosimilar are retained mostly by PBMs and third party payers and are not passed on to the patient. Because an approved biosimilar has equivalent efficacy and comparable safety with its reference product, a patient may derive no additional benefit from being treated with a biosimilar in place of its reference product unless he or she shares at least a portion of the cost savings.

POTENTIAL BENEFITS OF BIOSIMILARS

The justification for biosimilars is that the potential risk to an individual patient of switching to a lower-cost biosimilar should be outweighed by the potential benefit to society of expanding access to care for all.[43] Biosimilars should be more readily available to patients for whom the reference product had been inaccessible. Lower-priced biosimilars should introduce market competition, driving down the price of the reference product. The existence of multiple biosimilars of the same reference product should reduce not only the price of the reference product but also those of the biosimilars. Thus, the availability of biosimilars should decrease the cost of treating patients.

Given that a biosimilar should have equivalent efficacy and comparable safety with its reference product, the advantage of a biosimilar should be lower cost.[43] If a patient transitions from a reference product to its biosimilar to achieve cost savings, he or she should derive some personal benefit from this change. Unless the patient receives some monetary benefit by changing to the biosimilar, he or she most likely would prefer to continue taking the reference product. If only the payor saves money by requiring this "nonmedical switch," there is no incentive for a patient to comply with the change. Thus, patients should be able to obtain a biosimilar at a lower "out-of-pocket" cost than that for the reference product, with a minimal or waived copayment. Similarly, health care providers could be encouraged to prescribe lower-cost biosimilars by reducing or eliminating the requirement for prior authorization.

Although one would expect that more market competition should result in significant price reductions, with direct savings derived from use of a biosimilar instead of its reference product, market forces in the United States have not brought about price reductions for biosimilars that are of comparable magnitude with those in Scandinavian and other countries.

A patient receives effective therapy, whether treated with a biosimilar or its reference product. Even if the actual cost of a biosimilar is higher than that of its reference product, the introduction of the biosimilar likely provoked reduction of the reference product's price. As a result of this market competition, patients can obtain the prescribed biologic agent (either reference product or biosimilar) at a price lower than the former price of the reference product before entry of the biosimilar to the market. Thus, the availability of biosimilars should yield a net cost savings for the health care system and may improve treatment outcomes by expanding access to effective medications for more patients.[43] However, if PBMs and payors designate lower-priced reference products as being preferred over their biosimilars, market competition will be stifled. Then, if biosimilar manufacturers cannot gain market share and withdraw from the market, the prices of reference products likely will rise to their former levels or higher.[44] Thus, use of biosimilars should be encouraged to preserve a competitive market and sustain the availability of affordable medications for patients.

REFERENCES

1. Biologics Price Competition and Innovation Act of 2009, United States Code. Public Law 111–148, 124 Stat. 119, §7001-7003. Available at: https://www.congress.gov/111/plaws/publ148/PLAW-111publ148.pdf. Accessed May 9, 2019.
2. US Food and Drug Administration. Biosimilar product information. 2019. Available at: https://www.fda.gov/drugs/biosimilars/biosimilar-product-information. Accessed May 9, 2019.
3. Kay J, Schoels MM, Dorner T, et al. Consensus-based recommendations for the use of biosimilars to treat rheumatological diseases. Ann Rheum Dis 2018;77(2):165–74.
4. Mellstedt H, Niederwieser D, Ludwig H. The challenge of biosimilars. Ann Oncol 2008;19(3):411–9.
5. US Food & Drug Administration. Guidance for industry. Scientific considerations in demonstrating biosimilarity to a reference product. 2015. Available at: http://https://www.fda.gov/media/82647/download. Accessed May 9, 2019.
6. Park W, Yoo DH, Miranda P, et al. Efficacy and safety of switching from reference infliximab to CT-P13 compared with maintenance of CT-P13 in ankylosing spondylitis: 102-week data from the PLANETAS extension study. Ann Rheum Dis 2017;76(2):346–54.
7. Tanaka Y, Yamanaka H, Takeuchi T, et al. Safety and efficacy of CT-P13 in Japanese patients with rheumatoid arthritis in an extension phase or after switching from infliximab. Mod Rheumatol 2017;27(2):237–45.
8. Yoo DH, Prodanovic N, Jaworski J, et al. Efficacy and safety of CT-P13 (biosimilar infliximab) in patients with rheumatoid arthritis: comparison between switching

from reference infliximab to CT-P13 and continuing CT-P13 in the PLANETRA extension study. Ann Rheum Dis 2017;76(2):355–63.
9. Gerdes S, Thaci D, Griffiths CEM, et al. Multiple switches between GP2015, an etanercept biosimilar, with originator product do not impact efficacy, safety and immunogenicity in patients with chronic plaque-type psoriasis: 30-week results from the phase 3, confirmatory EGALITY study. J Eur Acad Dermatol Venereol 2018;32(3):420–7.
10. Poetzl J, Arlt I, von Richter O, et al. State-of-the-art immunogenicity evaluation in phase 3 confirmatory study (EGALITY) with etanercept biosimilar GP2015. J Eur Acad Dermatol Venereol 2018;32(4):e130–2.
11. Papp K, Bachelez H, Costanzo A, et al. Clinical similarity of the biosimilar ABP 501 compared with adalimumab after single transition: long-term results from a randomized controlled, double-blind, 52-week, phase III trial in patients with moderate-to-severe plaque psoriasis. Br J Dermatol 2017;177(6):1562–74.
12. Cohen SB, Alonso-Ruiz A, Klimiuk PA, et al. Similar efficacy, safety and immunogenicity of adalimumab biosimilar BI 695501 and Humira reference product in patients with moderately to severely active rheumatoid arthritis: results from the phase III randomised VOLTAIRE-RA equivalence study. Ann Rheum Dis 2018;77(6):914–21.
13. Smolen JS, Choe JY, Prodanovic N, et al. Safety, immunogenicity and efficacy after switching from reference infliximab to biosimilar SB2 compared with continuing reference infliximab and SB2 in patients with rheumatoid arthritis: results of a randomised, double-blind, phase III transition study. Ann Rheum Dis 2018;77(2):234–40.
14. Blauvelt A, Lacour JP, Fowler JF Jr, et al. Phase III randomized study of the proposed adalimumab biosimilar GP2017 in psoriasis: impact of multiple switches. Br J Dermatol 2018;179(3):623–31.
15. Kozlowski S, Woodcock J, Midthun K, et al. Developing the nation's biosimilars program. N Engl J Med 2011;365(5):385–8.
16. Emery P, Vencovsky J, Sylwestrzak A, et al. A phase III randomised, double-blind, parallel-group study comparing SB4 with etanercept reference product in patients with active rheumatoid arthritis despite methotrexate therapy. Ann Rheum Dis 2017;76(1):51–7.
17. Bridges SL Jr, White DW, Worthing AB, et al. The science behind biosimilars: entering a new era of biologic therapy. Arthritis Rheumatol 2018;70(3):334–44.
18. Schneider CK. Biosimilars in rheumatology: the wind of change. Ann Rheum Dis 2013;72(3):315–8.
19. Schiestl M, Stangler T, Torella C, et al. Acceptable changes in quality attributes of glycosylated biopharmaceuticals. Nat Biotechnol 2011;29(4):310–2.
20. Kim S, Song J, Park S, et al. Drifts in ADCC-related quality attributes of Herceptin®: impact on development of a trastuzumab biosimilar. MAbs 2017;9(4):704–14.
21. US Food & Drug Administration. FDA briefing document: Arthritis Advisory Committee meeting, February 09, 2016. BLA 125544: CT-P13, a proposed biosimilar to Remicade® (infliximab), Celltrion. 2016. Available at: https://www.fda.gov/media/95987/download. Accessed May 9, 2019.
22. Jørgensen KK, Olsen IC, Goll GL, et al. Switching from originator infliximab to biosimilar CT-P13 compared with maintained treatment with originator infliximab (NOR-SWITCH): a 52-week, randomised, double-blind, non-inferiority trial. Lancet 2017;389(10086):2304–16.

23. Glintborg B, Sorensen IJ, Loft AG, et al. A nationwide non-medical switch from originator infliximab to biosimilar CT-P13 in 802 patients with inflammatory arthritis: 1-year clinical outcomes from the DANBIO registry. Ann Rheum Dis 2017;76(8):1426–31.
24. Tweehuysen L, van den Bemt BJF, van Ingen IL, et al. Subjective complaints as the main reason for biosimilar discontinuation after open-label transition from reference infliximab to biosimilar infliximab. Arthritis Rheumatol 2018;70(1):60–8.
25. Tweehuysen L, Huiskes VJB, van den Bemt BJF, et al. Open-label, non-mandatory transitioning from originator etanercept to biosimilar SB4: six-month results from a controlled cohort study. Arthritis Rheumatol 2018;70(9):1408–18.
26. GaBI online - Generics and Biosimilars Initiative. Biosimilars approved in Europe. 2018. Available at: http://www.gabionline.net/Biosimilars/General/Biosimilars-approved-in-Europe. Accessed May 9, 2019.
27. QuintilesIMS. The impact of biosimilar competition in Europe. London (United Kingdom): QuintilesIMS; 2017. p. 1–33. Available at: https://www.medicinesforeurope.com/wp-content/uploads/2017/05/IMS-Biosimilar-2017_V9.pdf. Accessed May 9, 2019.
28. Mack A. Norway, biosimilars in different funding systems. What works? GaBi J 2015;4(2):90–2.
29. Brennan Z. AbbVie sees 80% discounts in Nordic market with new Humira biosimilars. 2018. Available at: https://www.raps.org/news-and-articles/news-articles/2018/11/abbvie-sees-80-discounts-in-nordic-market-with-ne. Accessed May 9, 2019.
30. GaBI Online - Generics and Biosimilars Initiative. Huge discount on biosimilar infliximab in Norway. 2015. Available at: http://www.gabionline.net/Biosimilars/General/Huge-discount-on-biosimilar-infliximab-in-Norway. Accessed May 9, 2019.
31. Berkrot B, Lee SY, Hirschler B. Merck, Samsung Bioepis launch discounted U.S. Remicade alternative. Reuters Health News. 2017. Available at: https://www.reuters.com/article/us-samsung-bioepis-johnson-johnson-remic/merck-samsung-bioepis-launch-discounted-u-s-remicade-alternative-idUSKBN1A91GL. Accessed May 9, 2019.
32. Rockoff JD. Behind the push for high-price EpiPen. Wall St J. August 7, 2017.
33. Wapner J. Understanding the hidden villain of Big Pharma: pharmacy benefit managers. Newsweek. 2017. Available at: http://www.newsweek.com/big-pharma-villain-pbm-569980. Accessed May 9, 2019.
34. Fiebach HR, Milne RA, Gallagher MJ, et al. Complaint: Pfizer Inc. v. Johnson & Johnson and Janssen Biotech, Inc. 2017. Available at: https://www.courtlistener.com/recap/gov.uscourts.paed.534730.1.0.pdf. Accessed May 9, 2019.
35. Smolen JS, Landewe R, Bijlsma J, et al. EULAR recommendations for the management of rheumatoid arthritis with synthetic and biological disease-modifying antirheumatic drugs: 2016 update. Ann Rheum Dis 2017;76(6):960–77.
36. US Centers for Medicare & Medicaid Services. Medicare Part B drug average sales price. 2018. Available at: https://www.cms.gov/medicare/medicare-fee-for-service-part-b-drugs/mcrpartbdrugavgsalesprice/index.Html. Accessed May 9, 2019.
37. US Centers for Medicare & Medicaid Services. Part B biosimilar biological product payment and required modifiers. 2018. Available at: https://www.cms.gov/Medicare/Medicare-Fee-for-Service-Part-B-Drugs/McrPartBDrugAvgSalesPrice/Part-B-Biosimilar-Biological-Product-Payment.html. Accessed May 9, 2019.

38. US Centers for Medicare & Medicaid Services. Medicare Part B drug average sales price: ASP drug pricing files April 2019 update. 2019. Available at: https://www.cms.gov/Medicare/Medicare-Fee-for-Service-Part-B-Drugs/McrPartBDrugAvgSalesPrice/2019ASPFiles.html. Accessed May 9, 2019.
39. Celltrion and Hospira have launched Inflectra® in U.S. Big Molecule Watch. 2016. Available at: https://www.bigmoleculewatch.com/2016/12/08/inflectra-launched-in-us/. Accessed May 9, 2019.
40. Stanton D. Discount dancers: Pfizer's infliximab matching Merck's new biosimilar rival. BioPharma-Reporter.com. 2017. Available at: https://www.biopharma-reporter.com/Article/2017/07/26/Pfizer-cuts-biosimilar-price-to-match-Merck-s-new-infliximab-rival. Accessed May 9, 2019.
41. Rockoff JD. Pfizer files antitrust lawsuit against J&J. Wall St J. September 21, 2017.
42. Merck Announces U.S. Launch of RENFLEXIS™ (infliximab-abda), a biosimilar of remicade, for all eligible indications. Kenilworth (NJ): Merck & Co., Inc; 2017. Available at: https://investors.merck.com/news/press-release-details/2017/Merck-Announces-US-Launch-of-RENFLEXIS-infliximab-abda-a-Biosimilar-of-Remicade-for-All-Eligible-Indications/default.aspx. Accessed May 9, 2019.
43. Kay J. Editorial: Biosimilars: new or déjà vu? Arthritis Rheumatol 2016;68(5):1049–52.
44. Rockoff JD. Knockoffs of biotech drugs bring paltry savings. Wall St J. May 5, 2016.

Printed and bound by CPI Group (UK) Ltd, Croydon, CR0 4YY
08/05/2025
01864747-0005